Interventions for Cardiovascular Disease

Editors

LEANNE H. FOWLER
JESSICA LANDRY

CRITICAL CARE NURSING CLINICS OF NORTH AMERICA

www.ccnursing.theclinics.com

Consulting Editor
JAN FOSTER

March 2019 • Volume 31 • Number 1

ELSEVIER

1600 John F. Kennedy Boulevard • Suite 1800 • Philadelphia, Pennsylvania, 19103-2899

http://www.theclinics.com

CRITICAL CARE NURSING CLINICS OF NORTH AMERICA Volume 31, Number 1
March 2019 ISSN 0899-5885, ISBN-13: 978-0-323-65483-8

Editor: Kerry Holland
Developmental Editor: Laura Fisher

Critical Care Nursing Clinics of North America (ISSN 0899-5885) is published quarterly by Elsevier Inc., 360 Park Avenue South, New York, NY 10010-1710. Months of issue are March, June, September, and December. Business and Editorial Offices: 1600 John F. Kennedy Blvd., Suite 1800, Philadelphia, PA 19103-2899. Periodicals postage paid at New York, NY and additional mailing offices. Subscription prices are $160.00 per year for US individuals, $406.00 per year for US institutions, $100.00 per year for US students and residents, $206.00 per year for Canadian individuals, $510.00 per year for Canadian institutions, $230.00 per year for international individuals, $510.00 per year for international institutions and $115.00 per year for Canadian and international students/residents. To receive student/resident rate, orders must be accompanied by name of affiliated institution, data of term, and the *signature* of program/residency coordinator on institution letterhead. Orders will be billed at individual rate until proof of status is received. Foreign air speed delivery is included in all *Clinics* subscription prices. All prices are subject to change without notice. **POSTMASTER:** Send address changes to *Critical Care Nursing Clinics of North America*, Elsevier Health Sciences Division, Subscription Customer Service, 3251 Riverport Lane, Maryland Heights, MO 63043. **Customer Service: 1-800-654-2452 (US and Canada); 314-447-8871 (outside US and Canada). Fax: 314-447-8029. E-mail:** JournalsCustomerService-usa@elsevier.com **(for print support) and** JournalsOnlineSupport-usa@elsevier.com **(for online support).**

Reprints. For copies of 100 or more of articles in this publication, please contact the Commercial Reprints Department, Elsevier Inc., 360 Park Avenue South, New York, New York, 10010-1710; Tel.: 212-633-3874, Fax: 212-633-3820, and E-mail: reprints@elsevier.com.

Critical Care Nursing Clinics of North America is covered in *MEDLINE/PubMed (Index Medicus), International Nursing Index, Nursing Citation Index, Cumulative Index to Nursing and Allied Health Literature,* and *RNdex Top 100.*

Contributors

CONSULTING EDITOR

JAN FOSTER, PhD, APRN, CNS
Formerly, Associate Professor, College of Nursing, Texas Woman's University,
Houston, Texas; Currently, President, Nursing Inquiry and Intervention, Inc,
The Woodlands, Texas

EDITORS

LEANNE H. FOWLER, DNP, MBA, APRN, AGACNP-BC, CNE
Assistant Professor of Clinical Nursing, Director of NP Programs, Program Coordinator,
AGACNP Concentration, LSU Health New Orleans School of Nursing, New Orleans,
Louisiana

JESSICA LANDRY, DNP, FNP-BC
Instructor of Clinical Nursing, Program Coordinator, PCFNP Concentration, LSU Health
New Orleans School of Nursing, New Orleans, Louisiana

AUTHORS

MELISSA A. BURMEISTER, PhD
Assistant Professor, Department of Pharmaceutical Sciences, William Carey University
School of Pharmacy, Biloxi, Mississippi

BENITA N. CHATMON, PhD, MSN, RN
Instructor of Clinical Nursing, School of Nursing, LSU Health New Orleans, New Orleans,
Louisiana

LATANJA LAWRENCE DIVENS, PhD, DNP, APRN, FNP-BC
Assistant Professor of Clinical Nursing, School of Nursing, LSU Health New Orleans,
New Orleans, Louisiana

JAMES FOLEY, MSN-HCSM, RN
Instructor, School of Nursing, LSU Health New Orleans, New Orleans, Louisiana

LEANNE H. FOWLER, DNP, MBA, APRN, AGACNP-BC, CNE
Assistant Professor of Clinical Nursing, Director of NP Programs, Program Coordinator,
AGACNP Concentration, LSU Health New Orleans School of Nursing, New Orleans,
Louisiana

ABIY HABTEWOLD, PhD
Assistant Professor, Department of Pharmaceutical Sciences, William Carey University
School of Pharmacy, Biloxi, Mississippi

DEEDRA H. HARRINGTON, DNP, MSN, APRN, ACNP-BC
Assistant Professor, BSN Coordinator, University of Louisiana at Lafayette, College of
Nursing and Allied Health Professions, Cardiology Intensivist Nurse Practitioner, Heart
Hospital of Lafayette, Lafayette, Louisiana

JESSICA L. JOHNSON, PharmD, BCPS
Associate Professor, Department of Pharmacy Practice and Administration, William
Carey University School of Pharmacy, Biloxi, Mississippi

JESSICA LANDRY, DNP, FNP-BC
Instructor of Clinical Nursing, Program Coordinator, PCFNP Concentration, LSU Health
New Orleans School of Nursing, New Orleans, Louisiana

NANETTE LeBLANC-MORALES, DNP, NP-C
Instructor of Nursing, Graduate Program, School of Nursing, LSU Health Sciences Center
– New Orleans, New Orleans, Louisiana

SUSAN LEE, RN, APRN, FNP-BC
Critical Care Nursing Instructor, School of Nursing, LSU Health New Orleans,
New Orleans, Louisiana

CHRISTY McDONALD LENAHAN, DNP, APRN, FNP-BC, ENP-C, CNE
Assistant Professor, Graduate Faculty Coordinator, University of Louisiana at Lafayette,
College of Nursing and Allied Health Professions, Lafayette, Louisiana

JENNIFER MARTIN, DNP, CRNA
Instructor of Clinical Nursing, Nurse Anesthesia Program, LSU Health New Orleans
School of Nursing, New Orleans, Louisiana

SHERRY L. RIVERA, DNP, ANP-C
Instructor of Clinical Nursing, Nurse Practitioner Program, LSU Health New Orleans
School of Nursing, New Orleans, Louisiana

TROY J. SMITH, PharmD
Assistant Professor, Department of Pharmacy Practice and Administration, William Carey
University School of Pharmacy, Biloxi, Mississippi

FRANCES STUEBEN, DNP, MSN, RN, CCRN, CHSE
Second Semester Senior Coordinator, Instructor, University of Louisiana at Lafayette,
College of Nursing and Allied Health Professions, Lafayette, Louisiana

SABRINA M. WHITE, DNP, APRN, ACNP-BC, CHFN
Heart Failure Nurse Practitioner, Department of Cardiology, East Jefferson General
Hospital, Metairie, Louisiana

LUCRETIA M. WILTZ-JAMES, MSN, APRN, FNP-BC
Clinical Instructor of Nursing Graduate Program, LSU Health New Orleans School of
Nursing, LSU Health Sciences Center, New Orleans, Louisiana

MONIQUE YOUNG, ACNP-BC
Staff Advanced Practitioner, Louisiana Heart Center, Slidell, Louisiana

Contents

Heart failure is a complex disease that interacts with other organ systems, such as the lungs, kidneys, and the liver, in a complex manner. The stages of heart failure often define the acuity and onset of disease symptoms and progression as well as treatment measures, in addition to the patient's functional class. As the neurohormonal and compensatory mechanisms become resistant and fail guideline-directed medical therapy, more advanced therapies are required. This article outlines treatments for advanced heart failure and provides a review of guideline-directed medical therapies leading into the late stages of heart failure.

This update presents evidence for new antiplatelet therapies including modified $P2Y_{12}$ inhibitors and a new class of thromboxane antagonists. Discussed are emerging data on established antihyperlipidemic medications that support an additional antiplatelet effect. Current information about the effectiveness of several bleeding reversal agents is discussed, and the concept of personalized antiplatelet therapy, wherein selection of an antiplatelet therapy is based on genetic factors or laboratory testing that predict response to therapy and risk of adverse effects. Finally, future drug targets are introduced and drug interactions that can be leveraged to design more effective and safe antiplatelet therapies are described.

Valvular heart dysfunction (VHD) affects up to 7% of adults up to age 44 year, whereas up to 13% of individuals older than 75 years are affected. The broad term of valvular heart disease includes dysfunction of one or more of the 4 heart valves, including the pulmonary valve, tricuspid valve, mitral valve, or aortic valve. Specifically the more frequent anomalies, implication, assessment, and treatment that will be described more extensively include aortic regurgitation, aortic stenosis, mitral regurgitation, or tricuspid regurgitation. The most prevalent cause of valvular heart disease stems from calcification and stiffening of the valve leaflets contributing to stenosis.

Peripheral disease affects both arteries and veins and encompasses pathophysiologic conditions that affect arterial, venous, and lymphatic circulations. This article discusses disorders of peripheral vascular disease (PVD) that affect the lower extremity. PVD is an obstruction in the arteries known as arteriosclerosis obliterans, a condition that manifests from insufficient tissue perfusion that results in hardening of the arteries. Peripheral artery disease leads to an inflammatory condition called atherosclerosis. People at greatest risk include smokers, diabetics, those with high blood pressure, and those with elevated cholesterol levels.

Hypertension is the most common primary diagnosis in the United States. Multiple sequelae of disease states are attributable to hypertension. Minimal to modest improvements in blood pressure can result in improved cardiovascular-related health outcomes. Despite the wealth of information available regarding the management and treatment of hypertension, the widespread control of hypertension continues to be an elusive challenge. A collaborative effort between patient and clinician using a balance of pharmacologic and nonpharmacologic interventions is essential to effectively manage and treat hypertension to avoid target organ damage. Prevention of acute organ damage related to hypertensive emergencies demands immediate intervention.

There is a well-established body of evidence that connects particular dietary lifestyle choices to good health. Despite this knowledge, rates of obesity, cardiovascular disease, and metabolic disease continue to rise. Culinary medicine uses what is known about the pharmacologic properties of food to treat, manage, and prevent disease. It fuses medicinal nutrition with culinary knowledge to help individuals adopt a diet that supports good health. Culinary techniques used to change behaviors and improve eating habits is an innovative modality to preserve and promote the health of a nation in need of effective medical interventions.

CRITICAL CARE NURSING
CLINICS OF NORTH AMERICA

FORTHCOMING ISSUES

June 2019
Quality Outcomes and Costs
Deborah Garbee and Denise Danna,
Editors

September 2019
Cardiothoracic Surgical Critical Care
Bryan Boling, *Editor*

December 2019
Psychological Issues in the ICU
Deborah W. Chapa, *Editor*

RECENT ISSUES

December 2018
Neonatal Nursing
Beth C. Diehl, *Editor*

September 2018
Sepsis
Jennifer B. Martin and
Jennifer E. Badeaux, *Editors*

June 2018
**Human Factors and Technology
in the ICU**
Shu-Fen Wung, *Editor*

SERIES OF RELATED INTEREST

Nursing Clinics of North America
http://www.nursing.theclinics.com

THE CLINICS ARE AVAILABLE ONLINE!
Access your subscription at:
www.theclinics.com

Preface

Improving Cardiovascular Health

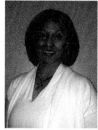 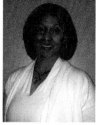

Leanne H. Fowler, DNP, MBA, AGACNP-BC, CNE   Jessica Landry, DNP, FNP-BC
Editors

Cardiovascular disease (CVD) is the leading cause of death in the United States across all races and ethnicities. The prevalence of CVD also increases with age despite gender. One in every four deaths is secondary to CVD, and coronary artery disease is the leading type of CVD, killing more than 366,000 yearly. Heart failure is the leading cause of poor quality of life, one of the leading causes of disability, and one of the most costly illnesses affecting Americans. Billions of dollars are spent annually for patients hospitalized with cardiovascular-related illness. Although primary and secondary preventative health promotion strategies are slowly reducing risks for CVD or recurrent acute illness, individuals with chronic illness, with low access to health care resources, and/or of low socioeconomic status are not benefiting and contribute to persistent health care burdens. Almost half of all Americans have at least one risk factor for CVD. As first-line clinicians, nursing professionals are in a unique position to contribute to the reduction of CVD, cardiovascular-related deaths, and overall health care burdens.

Critically ill patients suffering from cardiovascular illness are a particularly vulnerable population within hospitals and are at a high risk for increased morbidity, poor quality of life, and death. In addition, families of patients suffering critical cardiovascular illness also suffer and share the burdens of costly health care. Critical care nurses are uniquely positioned to positively impact the patient and family during health care delivery. Increased knowledge of therapeutic cardiovascular interventions can improve patient outcomes, deliver family-centered care, reduce health care costs, and

Crit Care Nurs Clin N Am 31 (2019) ix–x
https://doi.org/10.1016/j.cnc.2018.12.001
0899-5885/19/© 2018 Published by Elsevier Inc.

ultimately improve the cardiovascular health or the quality of life of individuals and families when implementing behavioral, medical, and surgical interventions for CVD.

Leanne H. Fowler, DNP, MBA, AGACNP-BC, CNE
LSU Health New Orleans School of Nursing
1900 Gravier Street
New Orleans, LA 70112, USA

Jessica Landry, DNP, FNP-BC
LSU Health New Orleans School of Nursing
1900 Gravier Street
New Orleans, LA 70112, USA

E-mail addresses:
lfowle@lsuhsc.edu (L.H. Fowler)
jland7@lsuhsc.edu (J. Landry)

Evidence-based Strategies for Advanced Heart Failure

Sabrina M. White, DNP, APRN, ACNP-BC, CHFN*

KEYWORDS

- Heart failure • Inotrope therapy • Vasodilator therapy • Internal cardiac defibrillator
- Cardiac resynchronization therapy • Mechanical circulatory device
- Heart transplant • Palliative care

KEY POINTS

- Guideline-directed medical therapy should be administered to all patients with heart failure with a reduced ejection fraction. Heart failure with a preserved ejection fraction can utilize the same guideline-directed medical therapy but may include additional drugs which are not used in patients with a reduced ejection fraction.
- Neurohormonal responses become resistant to standard heart failure treatment, leading to advanced heart failure treatments. Patients with comorbidities such as end-stage renal disease, liver disease, irreversible lung disease, and peripheral vascular disease are contraindicated to advanced therapies and may progress to destination therapy or end-of-life care.
- End-of-life care should be addressed early in the diagnosis of heart failure to introduce the dialogue and concept of shared decision making, as well as making an early introduction to palliative care and the advent of hospice meeting the biopsychosocial and spiritual needs of the patients with heart failure and their families.

Heart failure (HF) affects approximately 5.7 million adults annually, with an estimated national cost of $30.7 billion each year.[1] About half of the patients who are newly diagnosed with HF die within the first 5 years of diagnosis. As a result of the growing cost of HF treatments and higher readmission rates for HF. Medicare initiated reimbursement penalties for facilities with readmission rates greater than the current national rate of 21.6% according to Hospitals Compare.[2]

In 2013, American Heart Association (AHA)/American College of Cardiology (ACC)[3] developed specific evidence-based guidelines for the management and treatment of HF. These guidelines were developed as a result of extensive research analysis from a national and global perspective and were updated in 2016 and 2017.[4,5] Newer

Disclosure: S.M. White is a speaker for Novartis Pharmaceutical on the drug Entresto.
Department of Cardiology, East Jefferson General Hospital, 4224 Houma Boulevard, Suite 530, Metairie, LA 70006, USA
* 5601 Wimbledon Ct, New Orleans, LA 70131.
E-mail address: sabrinaw38@cox.net

medications and advanced therapies are discussed in the guidelines and have improved care for the HF population, resulting in patients living longer and creating a growing older population. This article outlines HF and evidence-based strategies for the treatment of late stages of HF.

HEART FAILURE DEFINITION, STAGING, CLASSIFICATIONS, AND GUIDELINE-DIRECTED THERAPY

The ACC/AHA 2013[3] Guidelines for the Management of Heart Failure Executive Summary provided standardized guidelines and definitions of HF to include HF with reduced ejection fraction (HFrEF), HF with preserved ejection fraction (HFpEF), and borderline HF. HF as a result of any cause is classified in one of these categories. HFrEF includes those patients with an ejection fraction (EF) of less than 40%, HFpEF includes those with an EF of greater than 40%, borderline preserved EF includes those with an initial EF between 41% and 49%, and HFpEF improved includes those with an EF that was reduced but improved to greater than 40%. The recommended medical therapy depends on the patient-specific definition as well as the New York Heart classification (NYHC) and staging of HF.

The term goal-directed medical therapy was coined to describe recommended therapies for HF. Although research is still in progress for HFpEF, the recommendation depends on the cause of HF but includes the same drugs used to treat HFrEF as well as calcium channel blockers, which are not guideline-directed medical therapy (GDMT) for HFrEF. HF therapies target the compensatory mechanisms: sympathetic nervous system (β-blockers) and renin-angiotensin-aldosterone system (angiotensin-converting enzyme inhibitors [ACEIs], angiotensin II receptor–blockers [ARBs], and aldosterone inhibitors) (**Table 1**).[6] In addition to diuretics, standard medical therapy for those patients with HFrEF is inclusive of all the medical therapies listed earlier. Newer therapies were added to the ACC/AHA/HFSA 2016 "focus update on new pharmacological therapy for heart failure"[4] and include Entresto, which is a combination of a sacubitril, which is a neprilysin inhibitor, and valsartan, an angiotensin receptor blocker. Ivabradine, which decreases the heart rate in patients on maximum tolerated dosages of β-blockers, was also added. Patients who are not responding to standard medical therapy can be placed on digoxin as a last alternative. Bidil is used in select patients who meet specific criteria. According to Anand and Florea,[7] substantial evidence exist that endothelial dysfunction and impaired bioavailability of nitric oxide contribute to the pathophysiology of HF, and the V-HeFT (Vasodilator Heart Failure Trial) confirmed this theory. The A-HeFT (African American Heart Failure Trial) evaluated the benefits of Bidil in African Americans and reported a mortality benefit with the isosorbide hydralazine combination accompanied by regression of left ventricular remodeling.[7]

ADDITIONAL GUIDELINE-DIRECTED MEDICAL THERAPIES FOR HEART FAILURE

Recent data encourage the use of internal cardiac defibrillators (ICDs), cardiac resynchronization therapy (CRT), and revascularization such as percutaneous transluminal coronary angiography with stent placements and/or surgical interventions (valve repairs and coronary artery bypass graft) as indicated for treatment of HF. The 2013 Appropriate Use Criteria for Implantable Cardioverter-Defibrillators and Cardiac Resynchronization Therapy[8] and 2018 national coverage determination for implantable defibrillators provide guidelines for device eligibility.[9] The patient must have an evaluation of the left ventricular EF, which now includes the use of cardiac MRI. The ICD criteria now include shared

Table 1
Evidence-based medical strategies for heart failure

HFrEF Medication Clinical Trials				
ACEIs	**Consensus 1**	**SOLVD**	**V-HeFT II**	**Overture**
ARBs	Elite	Elite 2	CHARM alternative	CHARM added
Angiotensin Receptor Antagonist	RALES	EPHESUS	—	—
β-Blockers	PRECISE CIBIS	COPERNICUS CIBIS II	COMET —	MDC/MERIT HF —
Digitalis	DIG	—	—	—
CRT	COMPANION	CARE-HF	—	—
Defibrillator	SCD-HeFT	—	—	—
Entresto	Paradigm-HF trial	—	—	—
Corlanor	SHIFT Study	—	—	—
HF with Normal EF Medication Clinical Trials				
ACEIs	Pep-CHF	—	—	—
ARBs	CHARMED reserved	I-Preserve	—	—
Digitalis	DIG Ancillary	—	—	—
Angiotensin Receptor Antagonist	Top Cat	—	—	—
β-Blockers	SENIORS	—	—	—
Diuretics	HONG KONG	—	—	—

decision-making criteria, in addition to those with severe nonischemic dilated cardiomyopathy without the advent of sustained ventricular ($\geq$30 seconds) tachycardia or cardiac arrest as a result of a ventricular arrhythmia. The patient must also be on maximum tolerated GDMT for at least 3 months and meet indications for ICD therapy (**Box 1**).

The CRT criteria as noted in the 2012 focused update of the 2008 Guidelines for Device-Based Therapy of Cardiac Rhythm Abnormalities[10] identifies those patients with progressive left ventricular systolic dysfunction with clinical HF symptoms and electromechanical dissociation as the cause for diminishing effective left ventricular contractility. These patients have HFrEF and must meet indications for CRT therapy (**Box 2**).

Multiple clinical trial data have shown benefit by decreasing hospitalizations by 30% and mortality benefit of 24% to 36% per 2013 appropriate use criteria for ICD and CRT therapy. The criteria noted that the COMPANION and CARE-HF trials revealed benefits of using CRT that include a reduction in death rate by 36% and a reduction in the mortality by 36%. However, Galve and colleagues[11] noted that those patients who received CRT defibrillators had a reduction in the need for ICD therapy caused by associated improvements in their LVEFs.

ADVANCED HEART FAILURE

Advanced HF is defined by progression of symptoms and failure to stabilize a patients' hemodynamics while on GDMT using the NYHC and HF staging as noted

---

Box 1
Clinical indications for internal cardiac defibrillator therapy

1. The patient must have a history of sustained ventricular tachycardia or cardiac arrest related to ventricular fibrillation.

2. Patients with a myocardial infarction (MI) with an EF of less than or equal to 30% must meet NYHC IV criteria, have had a coronary artery bypass graft (CABG) or percutaneous coronary intervention (PCI) within the past 3 months, and have had an MI within the past 40 days or clinical findings suggesting the need for coronary revascularization.

3. Patients with severe ischemic dilated cardiomyopathy with an EF less than or equal to 35%, NYHC II to III without episodes of sustained ventricular tachycardia, or cardiac arrest–related ventricular fibrillation must also have had a CABG or PCI within the past 3 months, and MI within the past 40 days or clinical findings suggesting the need for coronary revascularization.

4. Patients with severe nonischemic dilated cardiomyopathy with an EF less than or equal to 35%, NYHC II to III without episodes of sustained ventricular tachycardia or cardiac arrest–related ventricular fibrillation must also have had a CABG or PCI within the past 3 months, and MI within the past 40 days or clinical findings suggesting the need for coronary revascularization.

5. Patients with genetic or familial predisposition who are at high risk of developing life-threatening tachyarrhythmias such as hypertrophic cardiomyopathy and long QT syndrome.

6. Patients who have ICDs that require replacement because of end of battery life or device and/or lead malfunction.

---

earlier. Lainscak and colleagues[12] referred to advanced HF as a syndrome requiring a resting left ventricle EF less than 35%, NYHC of III to IV, or a peak oxygen uptake (Vo_2) less than 14 mL/kg/min. Frequent hospitalizations, continued decline in clinical symptoms despite GDMT, and hyponatremia have also been noted as indicators of advanced HF. However, the staging is of utmost importance and does not change once the HF progress is a structural issue and symptomatic on maximum tolerated medical management. AbouEzzeddine and Redfield[13] identified stage A as patients who are asymptomatic and have risk factors but no HF

Box 2
Clinical indications for cardiac resynchronization therapy

1. In patients with an EF of less than or equal to 35%, a QRS duration greater than or equal to 150 milliseconds, left bundle branch block (LBBB) pattern, NYHC II to IV, and sinus rhythm, CRT with or without ICD is indicated.

2. In patients with an EF of less than or equal to 35%, a QRS duration greater than or equal to 0.12 seconds, NYHC II to IV with atrial fibrillation, CRT with or without ICD is a reasonable recommendation. However, the patient must be on optimal medical therapy.

3. In patients with an EF of less than or equal to 35%, ischemic HF, sinus rhythm, or LBBB and a QRS duration greater than or equal to 0.12 seconds, NYHC II to IV, and on optimal medical therapy but frequent dependence on ventricular pacing is present, CRT with or without ICD is a reasonable recommendation.

4. Patients with an EF of less than or equal to 30%, a QRS duration greater than or equal to 0.12 seconds, NYHC II to IV, on optimal medical therapy but undergoing implantation of a permanent pacemaker and/or ICD with anticipation of frequent dependence on ventricular pacing may be considered for CRT.

symptoms. Stage B patients include stage A as well as the development of structural heart disease. Stage C patients develop overt HF symptoms as shown by increased filling pressure preventing the heart from maintaining peripheral perfusion and ultimately neglecting the metabolic demands of the body. Stage IV patients are never able to achieve metabolic stability and rapidly decompensate, requiring more aggressive medical therapy. Automatic ICD and CRT treatment are often performed before achieving this level of medical resistance. Advanced therapies for the treatment of HF include intravenous vasodilator, inotrope therapy, ventricular assist device (VAD) therapy, heart transplant, and ultimately palliative care/hospice.

ADVANCED THERAPIES FOR ADVANCED HEART FAILURE

Advanced HFs requires that the patients meet specific criteria. This article reviews requirements set forth by Medicare for each therapy. All of the patients must meet the HF stage C and D criteria, along with NYHC III and IV, and must have failed therapy despite documented maximum tolerated medical therapy to receive reimbursement for advanced HF treatments. Some patients may temporarily improve, but in many cases advanced therapies should be discussed, especially if the patient has recurrent hospitalizations.

VASODILATOR THERAPY

Vasodilator therapy is indicated for those with refractory HF requiring assistance with afterload and preload reduction. The patients who qualify for vasodilator therapy are on diuretic therapy and continue to have increased filling pressures, low cardiac output, and afterload reduction for those with hypertension and refractory HF. The vasodilators provide both arterial and venous dilatation to achieve these goals. The drugs of choice are nitroprusside and nitroglycerin. A prospective, observational study reviewed 64 subjects with a mean age of 55 years, the objective being to assess the effects of nitroglycerin ointment on mean arterial pressure and systemic vascular resistance in the emergency department. The results revealed that the mean arterial pressure and the thoracic fluid content decreased following application of the nitroglycerin ointment. Hemodynamic parameters were reviewed at baseline, 30, 60, and 120 minutes after adjusting for age, sex, and final emergency department diagnosis of acute HF. The cardiac index, cardiac output, systemic vascular resistance, and stroke volume did not show change.[14] Current literature for nitroglycerin and nesiritide/Natrecor are bias because these drugs have been used in HF for some time. Rayner-Hartley and colleagues[15] published an update on the management of acute HF and cited Ho and colleagues'[16] findings, which reported results of a large retrospective cohort study examining the effects of nitrate administration on short-term and long-term survival in 11,078 Canadian patients. In a propensity-matched analysis, there was no improvement in survival among patients treated with nitrates. Nesiritide/Natrecor was also evaluated in the ASCEND-HF trial; this was a randomized study with 2007 patients who were randomized to nesiritide/Natrecor versus placebo. The study revealed no significant difference in symptom burden, 30-day mortality, or rehospitalization.[17] A pharmacologic review of nitrates as a treatment of acute HF[18] evaluated various clinical trials that evaluated the clinical safety and efficacy of nitroglycerin. A case for the early use of high-dose nitrates was made based on the literature available before 2007. The recommendations were based on the mechanism of action of nitrates and the effectiveness of using it early in decompensation, when dosed accordingly. Nitrates have proven to have a systemic vascular resistance, peripheral vascular resistance (PVR), blood pressure, intubation rates, and various other health-related parameters.

INOTROPE THERAPY

The goal of inotrope therapy (milrinone/Primacor and dobutamine/Dobutrex) is to improve myocardial contractility and cardiac output, and reduce afterload, therefore improving overall tissue perfusion. Inotropes, such as milrinone/Primacor and dobutamine/Dobutrex, act through beta-adrenergic receptor agonist and phosphodiesterase-3 enzyme inhibition.[15] Pulmonary arterial oxygen saturations (PA_{O_2}) are performed to evaluate tissue extraction during use of inotrope and other advanced therapies in the critical care setting. The PA_{O_2} provides a direct measurement and can sense earlier changes in the patient's condition. Inotrope therapy is a temporary measure to sustain these patients while exploring other treatment options. The options include destination therapy, which may be palliation to improve or sustain quality of life or a bridge to transplant. Although inotropes can also be used as an intermittent or continuous home infusion, the hemodynamic and clinical improvements are transient and are typically followed by a decline in cardiac function, limiting options for long-term therapy.[19] Medicare coverage criteria administered by external infusion pump requires that the patient has New York Heart Class III or IV HF, dosages within the lowest possible range to improve symptoms, hemodynamic parameters within 6 months before starting the home infusion, a cardiac index (CI) less than or equal to 2.2 L/min/m^2, or a pulmonary capillary wedge pressure (PCWP) of greater than or equal to 20 mm Hg before the infusion starts. Once the infusion begins, the following criteria must be met: the CI has to show an improvement of greater than 2.2 L/min/m^2 and/or a PCWP of at least a 20% decrease during the initial infusion. The goal for these drugs is to achieve the lowest possible dose to control symptoms and provide documentation of attempted weaning within the first 3 months of therapy.

SHORT-TERM LEFT VENTRICULAR ASSIST DEVICE THERAPY

The use of left VADs (LVADs) in advanced-stage HF is growing because people are living longer with medical therapies. The devices are categorized into short-term and long-term devices. The intra-aortic balloon pump (IABP), TandemHeart, and the Impella are the most common devices.

INTRA-AORTIC BALLOON PUMP

The underlying disorder, physician experience, and comfort with the device determine which device is used. The IABP is a device inserted percutaneously into the aorta that counterpulsates with the patient's heartbeat. One of the most important aspects of the pumps is timing, or synchronizing the action of the device with the cardiac cycle.[20] The IABP decreases the pressure in the left ventricle, therefore increasing stroke volume. A pilot study performed by Pfluecke and colleagues[21] evaluated cerebral blood flow in 36 subjects who received an IABP for cardiogenic shock and found IABP therapy improves cerebral blood flow by improving cardiac output, decreasing systemic vascular resistance, and improving microvascular perfusion and renal blood flow. The benefits of using the IABP are insertion with minimal difficulty, being least expensive, and its use for patients who do not require long-term intense hemodynamic support. Many IABPs are inserted at the bedside during rapid decompensation states such as cardiogenic shock.

THE TandemHeart AND IMPELLA

The TandemHeart and Impella devices are percutaneous assist devices, in contrast with the IABP. They are short-term devices that can be used in patients requiring greater and longer hemodynamic support than the IABP. Both devices are inserted in a cardiac catheterization laboratory and are typically used as a bridge to VAD therapy or heart transplant, after a procedure, and/or after a heart transplant in patients with cardiogenic shock. The TandemHeart device is a percutaneous inserted device with a continuous-flow centrifugal extracorporeal assist device withdrawing oxygenated blood from the left atrium and returning it to the femoral artery (**Fig. 1**). The device has a venous cannula inserted in the left atrium trans-septally and an arterial cannula

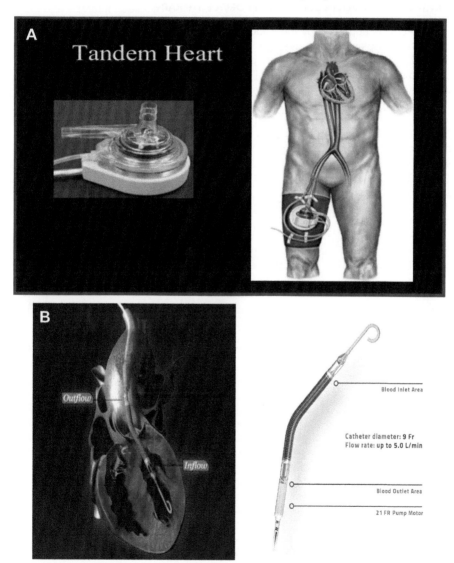

Fig. 1. Short-term VADs. (*A*) TandemHeart device. (*B*) Impella device. (*Courtesy of* [*A*] TandemLife, Pittsburgh, PA; with permission; and [*B*] Abiomed, Danvers, MA; with permission.)

inserted in the iliac-femoral artery. The Impella is a nonpulsatile microaxial-flow pump, placed across the aortic valve, and pumps blood from the left ventricle into the aorta in severe left ventricular dysfunction (see **Fig. 1**), Thereby unloading the left ventricle and reducing myocardial oxygen consumption and demand.[22] There are no specific Medicare criteria for insertion of these devices but the criteria and indications are similar to those discussed in relation to inotrope therapy, which allude to rapid deterioration and low output failure altering tissue perfusion. The decision to use either of the devices depends on the expertise of the physician inserting the device and the nurses caring for the patient.

LONG-TERM LEFT VENTRICULAR ASSIST DEVICE THERAPY

The LVAD was approved by the Food and Drug Administration (FDA) in 1990 as a bridge to transplant with an average VAD implant time of 108 days. The study was over a 7-year period and 95 patients participated, which allowed 75% of the participants to be transplanted.[23] Studies allowed for additional research to be performed, which eventually led to device improvement and clinical trials that explored the option of long-term therapy. According to Enciso,[2,23] 2300 orthotic heart transplants are performed each year, which does not nearly meet the requirements for 10% of the 6.6 million who need heart transplants in North America. The REMATCH trial later randomized patients to inotrope therapy versus LVAD therapy. The trial showed a good survival rate for patients randomized to LVAD therapy compared with inotropes at 1 year (52% vs 25%, $P = .002$) (Rose and colleagues[24]). As a result of the supply and demand for treatment options, the limited availability of heart transplants, and the success of the device in the trial, the FDA approved bridge to transplant and destination therapy.[24]

The Recommendations for the Use of Mechanical Circulatory Support: Ambulatory and Community Patient Care, Scientific Statement (2017)[25] focus on the most commonly used LVADs, which are the HeartWare centrifugal pump (**Fig. 2**) and the

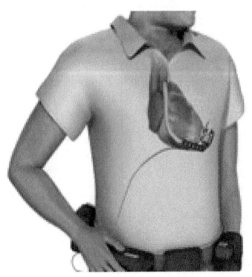

Fig. 2. Long-term VAD: HeartWare HVAD pump. (*Reproduced with permission of* Medtronic, Inc.)

HeartMate II axial flow pump (HeartMate II LVAS images can be viewed at http://www.thoratec.com/about-us/media-room/library.aspx). Regardless of which pump is chosen, both pumps help to empty the heart by assisting the blood flow from the left ventricle to the descending aorta. The cannula for both devices is attached directly to the left ventricle and the aorta. Long-term LVADs have no specific criteria for use under Medicare, but there are specific indications before implant.[26] Indications are the same as the criteria mentioned for inotrope therapy. In addition to the criteria for inotrope therapy, the transpulmonary gradient (TPG; ≤15 mm Hg), PVR (≤3 dyn*s/cm5), and the aortic valve should be evaluated. The TPG and PVR evaluate the function of the pulmonary gradient and right ventricle, which has to have normal function to receive an LVAD.[27] The overall incidence of right HF (RHF) can be as high as 30% in patients receiving an LVAD, with 71% of patients alive at 180 days compared with 89% of those without RHF.[23] In the event that the right ventricle fails, a right VAD or biventricular assist device may be inserted. There are additional clinical trials that support the use of the LVAD and HeartWare HVAD, which are the ADVANCE HVAD trial and the HeartMate II trial. The ADVANCE HVAD trial revealed that the HVAD device was noninferior to the HeartMate II device, with a 1-year survival of 86% and an enhanced quality of life (QOL) as seen with the HeartMate II. In the HeartMate II trial, the pulsatile flow device treatment was compared with continuous pulsatile flow treatment with the HeartMate II LVAD and patients treated with the HeartMate II had improved survival, significant reductions in adverse events, and improved QOL and functional capacity.[2,28] VADs offer an opportunity to improve survival and sustain quality of life across a spectrum of patients. In the advent of improving mechanical circulatory device therapy, some patients have shown improved heart function from resting the ventricle and their devices have been explanted.

ORTHOTIC HEART TRANSPLANT

Orthotic heart transplant (OHT) is recommended for patients who progress to stage D HF despite maximum tolerated GDMT, device therapy, and surgical management (ACCF/AHA, 2013)[29] All of the criteria listed for Medicare reimbursement of inotrope therapy and long-term device therapy are required for heart transplant consideration. The International Society for Heart and Lung Transplantation listing criteria 2006 were revised in 2016, and mainly concentrated on congenital heart disease, restrictive cardiomyopathy, and infectious disease. These areas were of interest to the committee and were not fully addressed in the previous update. A review of the 2006 guidelines was performed, focusing on new information and evolution in practice requiring change. The listing criteria for OHT did not change despite a review of practices (**Box 3**).[29]

Heart transplant is often the last recourse for patients who progress to end-stage HF. The goal is to keep the original organ as long as possible to prevent long-term effects of heart transplant, which include suppressing the immune system, predisposing the patient to opportunistic infection; medication-induced diabetes; and renal complications. There are contraindications to OHT as a result of not meeting the listing criteria requirements or evidence of irreversible multisystem organ failure. In the advent of new technology, patients not eligible for OHT may be evaluated by a multidisciplinary team for destination therapy with an LVAD depending on their ability to operate and care for the device.

PALLIATIVE CARE AND HOSPICE

The World Health Organization[30] defined palliative care as an approach that improves the QOL of patients and their families facing the problems associated with

---

Box 3
The International Society for Heart and Lung Transplantation listing criteria 2006

1. Cardiopulmonary stress test, which should be less than or equal to 14 without β-blocker therapy and less than or equal to 12 if the patient is on β-blocker therapy

2. HF prognostic scores using the Seattle Heart Failure Model of less than 80% or the Heart Failure Survival Score in the high/medium risk range

3. Diagnostic right heart catheterization every 3 to 6 months after listing

4. Evaluation of comorbidities and their implications for OHT, which includes the following: age, obesity, cancer, diabetes with end-organ damage, renal dysfunction, peripheral vascular disease, frailty, and severe symptomatic cerebral vascular disease

5. Evaluation of tobacco, substance abuse, and psychosocial evaluation

Data from Mehra MR, Canter CE, Hannan MM, et al. The 2016 International Society for Heart Lung Transplantation listing criteria for heart transplantation: a 10-year update. J Heart Lung Transplant 2016;35(1):1–23.

---

life-threatening illness, through the prevention and relief of suffering by means of early identification and accurate assessment and treatment of pain and other problems (physical, psychosocial, and spiritual). End-of-life discussion should begin at initial diagnosis, which introduces the advent of a disease that can be controlled initially but progresses over time. The medications controlling the neurohormonal cascade may not be sustained with GDMT or advanced therapies in advanced HF. Alder and colleagues[31] discussed shared decision making as a central focus in the care of chronic illnesses. Shared decision making involves establishing and fostering decisions among the patient, family and/or caregivers, and the medical team. Primary conversations should surround end-of-life measures, including whether the patient wants aggressive measures at end of life. If not, define what measures should be administered. Health care providers should have a systematic way of addressing end-of-life care for patients in advanced care, planning measures that incorporate the transition of palliative care to hospice. Often transition from end-stage HF to hospice is difficult and resistance may be met by both the patient and/or family members. Lemond and Allen[32] performed a literature review revealing the integration of palliative care as not being fully understood, and difficult prognostication combined with caregiver inexperience with end-of-life issues as contributors to barriers to integrating palliative care.

Palliative care often softens the transition, allowing the palliative care staff to interact with the family from a biopsychosocial perspective and assessing the more intricate needs, improving QOL by controlling chronic disease symptoms not prolonging life. In contrast with palliative care, hospice uses an interdisciplinary approach to deliver medical, social, physical, emotional, and spiritual services through the use of a broad spectrum of caregivers within the defined time frame at the end of life.[32] Eligibility for hospice must include the following: the patient must have Medicare part A, must be certified by a physician as being terminally ill, and must have a prognosis of 6 months or less if the disease runs its normal course. Hospice can be provided in the home or in an in-patient setting.[33]

SUMMARY

HF is defined as a clinical syndrome because of the complexity of the disease process. The classification of the stage and functional class of HF and treatment response to guideline-directed medical therapy often determine treatment measures. The patient's failed response to the neurohormonal cascade of treatments determines the advanced therapy and the diagnosis of late-stage or advanced HF. The choice of late-stage or advanced HF treatment versus palliative care or hospice depends on the patient's comorbidities. There are various reasons to make the choice of advanced treatment versus palliative care or hospice, but each decision is individualized and should be a shared decision between the patient, the patient's support system, and the medical team.

There is a definite need for research, as noted in the Paradigm-HF trial and the SHIFT Study which introduce 2 newer classes of drugs approved by the FDA within the last few years (Ivabradine and Entresto). Stem cell therapy for HF, also known as cardiopoietic stem cell therapy is presently in its research phase for treatment of chronic heart failure performed a prospective multi-center, randomized trial in which 319 patients were screened but only 48 patients were randomized.[34] The patients were randomized to standard of care alone which consisted of a beta blocker, ACE inhibitor or ARB and a diuretic versus standard of care and stem cell therapy. There was no evidence of toxicity in the stem cell arm but the LVEF was improved (from 27.5 to 34.5%) versus standard of care alone (from 27.8 to 28%) and there was a reduction in the left ventricular end systolic volume. The stem cell therapy group also had improvements in their 6 minute walk test, NYHC functional status, quality of life, physical performance, overall survival and decreased hospitalizations. cardiopoietic stem cell therapy was found feasible and safe with signs of benefit in the management of chronic heart failure despite the small sample size.

REFERENCES

1. Centers for Disease Control and Prevention. Heart failure fact sheet. Available at: http://www.cdc.gov/DHDSP/data_statistics/fact_sheets/fs_heart_failure.htm. ND. Accessed April 30, 2018.
2. Hospitals Compare. Rate of unplanned readmission for heart failure. Available at: https://www.medicare.gov/hospitalcompare. ND. Accessed April 30, 2018.
3. 2013 ACCF/AHA guidelines for the management of heart failure: executive summary: a report of the American College of Cardiology Foundation/American Heart Association task force on practice guidelines. 2013. Available at: http://content.onlinejacc.org/. Accessed May 1, 2018.
4. 2016 ACC/AHA/HFSA focused update on new pharmacological therapy for heart failure: an update of the 2013 ACCF/AHA guideline for the management of heart failure. 2016. Available at: http://content.onlinejacc.org/. Accessed May 1, 2018.
5. 2017 ACC/AHA/HFSA focused update on new pharmacological therapy for heart failure: an update of the 2013 ACCF/AHA guideline for the management of heart failure. 2016. Available at: http://content.onlinejacc.org/. Accessed May 1, 2018.
6. O'Donovan KO. Milrinone therapy in adults with heart failure. BJCardN 2013;8: 426–31.
7. Anand IS, Florea VG. Traditional and novel approaches to management of heart failure: successes and failures. Cardiol Clin 2008;26:59–72.
8. ACCF/HRS/AHA/ASE/HFSA/SCAI/SCCT/SCMR 2013 appropriate use criteria for implantable cardioverter defibrillators and cardiac synchronization therapy (2013). A report of the American College of Cardiology Foundation Appropriate Use Criteria, Heart Rhythm Society, American Heart Association, American Society of Echocardiography, Heart Failure Society of America, Society

for Cardiovascular Angiography and Interventions, Society of Cardiovascular Computed Tomography, and Society for Cardiovascular Magnetic Resonance (2013). 2013. Available at: http://content.onlinejacc.org/. Accessed May 15, 2018.

9. 2018 National coverage determination for implantable defibrillators. Decision memo for implantable cardioverter defibrillators (CAG-00157R4). (ND). Available at: https://www.cms.gov/medicare-coverage-database/details/nca-decision-memo.aspx?NCAId=288. ND. Accessed May 18, 2018.

10. 2012 ACCF/AHA/HRS focused update incorporated into the ACCF/AHA/HRS 2008 guidelines for device-based therapy of cardiac rhythm abnormalities (2012). A report of the American College of Cardiology Foundation/American Heart Association Task Force on Practice Guidelines and Heart Rhythm Society. 2012. Available at: http://content.onlinejacc.org/. Accessed May 18, 2018.

11. Galve E, Oristrell G, Acosta G, et al. Cardiac resynchronization therapy is associated with a reduction in ICD therapies as it improves ventricular function. Clin Cardiol 2018;41:803–8.

12. Lainscak M, Spoletini I, Coats A. Definition and classification of heart failure. Int Cardiovasc Forum J 2017;10:3–7.

13. AbouEzzeddine OF, Redfield MM. Who has advanced heart failure? Definition and epidemiology. Congest Heart Fail 2011;17(4):160–8.

14. Mumma BE, Dhingra K, Kurlinkus C, et al. Hemodynamic effects of nitroglycerin ointment in emergency departments patients. J Emerg Med 2014;47(2):192–7.

15. Rayner-Hartley E, Virani S, Toma M. Update on the management of acute heart failure. Curr Opin Cardiol 2018;33(2):225–31.

16. Ho EC, Parker JD, Austin PC, et al. Impact of nitrate use on survival in acute heart failure; a propensity matched analysis. J Am Heart Assoc 2016;5 [pii: e002531].

17. O'Connor CM, Starling RC, Hernandez AF, et al. Effects of nesiritide in patients with acute decompensated heart failure. N Engl J Med 2011;365:32–43.

18. Alzahri MS, Rohra A, Peacock FW. Pharmacological therapy: nitrates in the treatment of acute heart failure. Card Fail Rev 2016;2(1):51–5.

19. Ahmad T, Patel CB, Milano CA, et al. When the heart runs out of heartbeats: treatment options for refractory end stage heart failure. Circulation 2016;125:2948–55.

20. Hanlon-Pena PM, Quaal SJ. Intra-aortic balloon pump timing: review of evidence supporting current practice. Am J Crit Care 2011;20(4):323–33.

21. Pfluecke C, Christoph M, Kolschmann S, et al. Intra-aortic balloon pump (IABP) counterpulsation improves cerebral perfusion in patients with decreased left ventricular function. Perfusion 2014;29(6):511–6.

22. Peltran J, Oses P, Calderon J, et al. Impella 5.0 microaxial pump as a right ventricular assist device after surgical treatment of posterior post infarction ventricular septal defect. Perfusion 2014;29(5):472–6.

23. Enciso JS. Mechanical circulatory support: current status and future directions. Prog Cardiovasc Dis 2016;58:444–54.

24. Rose EA, Gelijns AC, Moskowitz AJ. Long-term use of a left ventricular assist device for end stage heart failure. N Engl J Med 2001;345(20):1435–42.

25. Cook JL, Colvin M, Francis GS. Recommendations for use of mechanical circulatory support: ambulatory and community patient care: a scientific statement from the American Heart Association. Circulation 2017;135:e1145–58. Available at: http://

circahajournals.org/content/early/2017/05/30/CIR. 0000000000000507.citation. Accessed May 22, 2018.

26. Miller LW, Guglin M. Patient selection for ventricular assist devices a moving target. J Am Coll Cardiol 2013;61(12):1209–21.
27. Gustafsson F, Rogers JG. Left ventricular assist device therapy in advance heart failure: patient selection and outcomes. Eur J Heart Fail 2017;19:595–602.
28. Birati EY, Jessup M. Left ventricular assist devices in the management of heart failure. Card Fail Rev 2015;1(1):25–30.
29. Mehra MR, Canter CE, Hannan MM, et al. The 2016 International Society for Heart Lung Transplantation listing criteria for heart transplantation: a 10-year update. 2016. Available at: https://doi.org/10.1016/j.healun.2015.10.023. Accessed June 1, 2018.
30. World Health Organization. WHO definition of palliative care. 2009. Available at: www.who.int/cancer/palliative/definition. Accessed May 30, 2018.
31. Adler ED, Judith Z, Goldfinger JZ, et al. Palliative care treatment of advanced heart failure. Circulation 2009;120:2597–606.
32. LeMond L, Allen LA. Palliative care and hospice in advanced heart failure. Prog Cardiovasc Dis 2011;54(2):168–78.
33. National Hospice and Palliative Care Organization (ND). Hospice Eligibility Requirements. Available at: https://www.nhpco.org/about/hospice-care.
34. Bartunek J, Behfar A, Dolatabadi D, et al. Cardiopoietic Stem Cell Therapy in Heart Failure. J Am ACC 2013;61(3):2329–38.

Cardiovascular Risk Reduction

A Pharmacotherapeutic Update for Antiplatelet Medications

Troy J. Smith, PharmD[a],*, Jessica L. Johnson, PharmD, BCPS[a],
Abiy Habtewold, PhD[b], Melissa A. Burmeister, PhD[b]

KEYWORDS

- Antiplatelet • Cardiovascular disease • Pharmacotherapy

KEY POINTS

- Platelets are activated by chemical signals binding to ADP, GPIIb/IIIa, and thromboxane receptors; each of these receptor pathways is a drug target for pharmacotherapy of cardiovascular disease.
- Novel antiplatelet therapies being developed include PPAR agonists, thromboxane receptor antagonists, and thromboxane synthesis inhibitors, and chemically modified $P2Y_{12}$ antagonists.
- Bleeding risk is estimated using comorbidity scoring tools. Bleeding reversal agents include platelet transfusion and novel monoclonal antibodies in development.
- Pharmacogenomic variation regulates gene expression of platelet receptors and drug metabolism, which can all affect safety and efficacy of pharmacotherapy and support precision medicine.
- Drug interactions can enhance or delay effects of antiplatelet therapies through impaired absorption or metabolism.

INTRODUCTION

The incidence of cardiovascular disease (CVD) in the United States has reached epidemic proportions. Although the rate of CVD death fell by 6.7% between 2004 and 2014, it remains the highest-ranking cause of death in the United States, accounting for approximately one in every three deaths from any cause.[1] An estimated 2200 Americans die from CVD-related complications daily, with millions of emergency department visits and critical care patient stays also associated with CVD.[1]

Disclosure Statement: The authors have nothing to disclose.
[a] Department of Pharmacy Practice and Administration, William Carey University School of Pharmacy, 19640 MS-67, Biloxi, MS 39532, USA; [b] Department of Pharmaceutical Sciences, William Carey University School of Pharmacy, 19640 MS-67, Biloxi, MS 39532, USA
* Corresponding author.
E-mail address: tjsmith@wmcarey.edu

Crit Care Nurs Clin N Am 31 (2019) 15–30
https://doi.org/10.1016/j.cnc.2018.11.001
0899-5885/19/© 2018 Elsevier Inc. All rights reserved.

Considering the significant morbidity and mortality linked to CVD and the economic burden of CVD on the workforce and health care system, it becomes critical to identify cost-effective and efficacious therapies for preventing and treating the disease and its related sequelae.[2]

Atherothrombosis is the common pathway underlying several related vasculopathies comprising the CVDs. These include acute coronary syndrome (ACS: unstable angina, myocardial infarction [MI]), cerebrovascular accident, coronary artery disease (CAD), and peripheral artery disease. Platelets become activated when collagen proteins bind to glycoprotein (GP) Ia/IIa and GPVI receptors located at the cell surface (**Fig. 1**). Activated platelets then change shape and release clotting mediators, which subsequently activate GPIIb/IIIa receptors to promote platelet aggregation. ADP, thromboxane A_2 (TXA2), and thrombin also trigger platelet activation through activation of G protein–coupled receptors. TXA2 is metabolized to TXB2, and thrombin enzymatically converts fibrinogen to fibrin. Through inhibition of these activation and aggregation processes, antiplatelet therapy has proven to be a mainstay in the prevention and treatment of CVD events.[3]

Three drug classes form a strong triad of antiplatelet therapy and are often used in varying combinations at different points in the disease process. Aspirin is the most widely used antiplatelet agent. Viewed by many as the first-line therapy, aspirin prevents the conversion of arachidonic acid (AA) to TXA2 through inhibition of platelet cyclooxygenase (COX) enzymes.[3] The highly successful $P2Y_{12}$ inhibitors prevent platelet aggregation by blocking the $P2Y_{12}$ receptor, which is a receptor for ADP. Often aspirin and $P2Y_{12}$ inhibitors are used together as a dual antiplatelet therapy (DAPT) regimen. GPIIb/IIIa inhibitors, which are most frequently used during

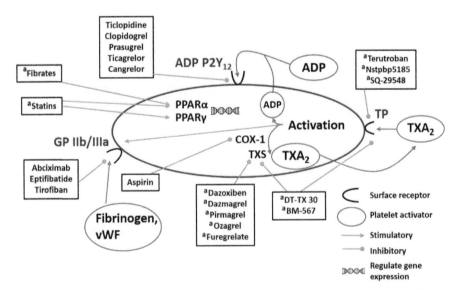

Fig. 1. Platelet activation pathways and antiplatelet medications. Three activation pathways for platelets include platelet surface receptors including the $P2Y_{12}$ ADP receptor, the thromboxane TP receptor, and the glycoprotein IIb/IIIa receptor. Antiplatelet drugs inhibit these receptors or inhibit the synthesis of platelet-activating chemicals that bind to these surface receptors. COX, cyclooxygenase; PPAR, peroxisome proliferator-activated receptor; TXA2, thromboxane A_2; TXS, thromboxane synthase; vWF, von Willebrand factor. [a]Investigational drug or novel target. (*Adapted from* Schafer AI. Antiplatelet therapy. Am J Med 1996;101(2):201; with permission.)

percutaneous coronary intervention (PCI), prevent platelet aggregation and thrombus formation by inhibiting the GPIIb/IIIa receptors on the surface of platelets. This article does not review the established evidence in support of these therapies but rather expands on updates to this well-known triad. Here we present studies from the past decade or so that examine novel drugs and dosage guidelines; explore new indications for old medications; and lay a foundation for potential future drug targets that are currently being tested in animal models. These new and investigational medications include intravenous formulations of the $P2Y_{12}$ inhibitors, the peroxisome proliferator-activator receptor (PPAR) agonists (ie, statins and fibrates), and thromboxane prostanoid (TP) receptor antagonists.

In line with the effort to continually improve patient care, guidelines for antiplatelet treatment regimen (ie, dosing, route of administration, timing and duration of administration, combination with other therapies) continue to develop as data from clinical trials and animal studies emerge. Cost-effectiveness and patient adherence significantly influence drug selection and health outcomes and should be considered. Although antiplatelet therapies significantly improve outcomes, patient response can also vary because of genetic factors that alter either drug metabolism[4–6] (eg, gene polymorphisms) or platelet reactivity.[7–9] The ultimate goal of pharmacotherapy in CVD is to identify those therapies that improve antiplatelet activity most effectively and exhibit the greatest antithrombotic effect without causing an unacceptable increase in hemorrhagic events. This update equips the critical care nurse to provide optimal, evidence-based care to patients presenting with CVD.

PHARMACOLOGY

Antiplatelet drugs exhibit varying pharmacokinetic (ie, what the body does to the drug; the time-course of a drug's absorption, bioavailability, distribution, metabolism, and excretion) and pharmacodynamic (ie, the study of how a drug affects an organism) properties, degrees of efficacy, and safety profiles, in part, because they are metabolized differently and function via different mechanisms of action. In the critical care setting, the choice of an antiplatelet agent is governed by cost, medication administration factors (ie, intravenous vs oral availability, need for rapid-acting agents), and patient response (ie, reduced risk of thrombotic events vs bleeding risk).

$P2Y_{12}$ Adenosine Diphosphate Receptor Inhibitors

There are five $P2Y_{12}$ inhibitors currently on the market in the United States: ticlopidine, clopidogrel, prasugrel, ticagrelor, and cangrelor (**Table 1**). These drugs reduce platelet aggregation by inhibiting the $P2Y_{12}$ receptor.[10] The $P2Y_{12}$ receptor is the main platelet receptor responsible for ADP-induced platelet aggregation via activation of GPIIb/IIIa receptors (see **Fig. 1**). Members of the thienopyridine drug class (ticlopidine, clopidogrel, and prasugrel), which are typically administered orally, indirectly and irreversibly inhibit the $P2Y_{12}$ subtype of the ADP receptor by covalently binding to it.[10]

Approved by the Food and Drug Administration (FDA) in 2015, intravenously administered cangrelor is the newest nonthienopyridine $P2Y_{12}$ inhibitor beneficial for ischemic events.[11] Cangrelor, which is chemically related to ticagrelor, has a high affinity for the $P2Y_{12}$ receptor, and the two drugs (unlike the thienopyridines clopidogrel, prasugrel, and ticlopidine) directly and reversibly inhibit the receptor by causing it to undergo a conformational change.[10] Cangrelor has been tested head-to-head against clopidogrel in PCI and demonstrates similar or slightly superior efficacy in prevention of cardiovascular events and stent thrombosis during the first 48 hours.[12] Because of the higher cost associated with a branded, intravenous drug formulation, cangrelor is

Table 1
P2Y$_{12}$ inhibitors used to treat cardiovascular disease

Drug	Route	FDA-Labeled Indications	Dosing	Reversible Receptor Binding?	Onset of Action	Duration of Action	Prodrug	Clinical Pearls
Ticlopidine (Ticlid)	PO	DVT prophylaxis	250 mg twice daily	No	48–72 h	7–10 d	No	Rarely used because of adverse effects
Clopidogrel (Plavix)	PO	ACS, recent MI, recent stroke, or PAD	300-mg LD, then 75 mg daily	No	2–6 h	3–10 d	Yes, CYP2C19	Greatest considerations for pharmacogenomics and drug interactions
Prasugrel (Effient)	PO	ACS	60-mg LD, then 10 mg daily	No	30 m	7–10 d	Yes, CYP2C19	Contraindicated in stroke and age >75
Ticagrelor (Brilinta)	PO	ACS or history of MI	180-mg LD, then 90 mg twice daily	Yes	30 m	3–5 d	No	Monitor digoxin levels
Cangrelor (Kengreal)	IV	Adjunct to PCI in P2Y$_{12}$-naive patients not taking a GPIIb/IIIa inhibitor	30-µg/kg LD bolus, then 4 µg/kg/min	Yes	2 m	1 h	No	Requires dedicated IV line

Abbreviations: DVT, deep vein thrombosis; IV, intravenous; LD, loading dose; PAD, peripheral artery disease; PO, oral.
Data from Refs. [10,11,13,76,88]

generally considered most useful for patients who cannot tolerate oral medications during the periprocedural loading dose timeframe. Cangrelor has also been investigated as a bridging agent for patients awaiting coronary bypass surgery, because of its reversibility and short offset. However, an FDA advisory committee recommended against this expanded indication citing a lack of supporting evidence.[13]

Should cangrelor be used in a clinical setting as a temporary, short-acting antiplatelet agent for patients with requiring PCI, the need would eventually arise for the patient to be switched to an oral agent after the first 24 to 48 hours of intravenous cangrelor therapy. The evidence supporting and exploring strategies to bridge from cangrelor to an oral agent is limited, but important, given cangrelor's quick reversibility and the delayed onset of effect of oral thienopyridines because of their comparatively slower absorption and need for hepatic bioactivation. An international expert consensus recommends administration of the oral agent immediately following discontinuation of the intravenous infusion of cangrelor to avoid any gap in antiplatelet effect.[14]

Peroxisome Proliferator-Activated Receptor Agonists

Statins and fibrates are primarily recognized for their antihyperlipidemic effects, whereby they lower serum cholesterol levels and prevent atherothrombosis and its related sequelae (eg, heart attack, stroke).[15] However, there is a growing body of evidence demonstrating pleiotropic effects of lipid-lowering drugs. With regards to reducing cardiovascular risk, they exhibit the added benefit of inhibiting platelet function and thrombosis/plaque rupture via mechanisms that occur independently from their cholesterol-lowering effect.[16–19]

The primary mechanism by which statins and fibrates elicit an antiplatelet effect is through activation of PPARs.[16] PPARs are a group of nuclear receptor phosphoproteins that function as transcription factors that regulate gene expression related to lipid and energy metabolism, inflammation, and atherosclerotic plaque formation (see **Fig. 1**).[20] Three types of PPARs have been identified: α, γ, and delta (Δ) (or β). Statins (eg, atorvastatin, simvastatin, pravastin, rosuvastatin) act as effective PPARα and PPARγ agonists, whereas fibrates (eg, fenofibrate, gemfibrozil, clofibrate, bezafibrate) selectively target PPARα.[16,21] Through their agonism at PPARα and PPARγ, statins reduce collagen- and ADP-mediated platelet aggregation by interfering with the signaling cascade required for platelet activation.[16,21] This mechanism of action is similar to that of the P2Y$_{12}$ inhibitors.

Two additional ways that statin therapy inhibits platelet activity is through interference of redox (ie, free radical) signaling and reduction of circulating levels of platelet-derived microparticles (PMPs). Free radicals include the reactive oxygen species superoxide, nitric oxide (NO), and hydrogen peroxide. Reactive oxygen species are unstable molecules that cause oxidative stress that is toxic to cells, DNA, and protein.[22] Reactive oxygen species also generate proaggregating molecules called isoprostanes.[22,23] Despite its cytotoxic effect, NO inhibits platelet activation and is a potent vasodilator.[24,25] Atorvastatin upregulates the expression of the enzyme responsible for producing NO[18,26] and inhibits an enzyme responsible for generating superoxide, resulting in the inhibition of platelet isoprostanes and TXA2.[27,28] PMPs are typically regarded as markers of platelet activity, and new evidence indicates that they also function as signaling molecules that facilitate crosstalk between inflammatory cells and the vasculature during CVD.[29] Increased levels of circulating PMPs are increasingly being linked to the pathogenesis of atherthrombosis.[29,30] Expression of the GPIIb/IIIa receptor on the surface of PMPs and thrombin-induced platelet activity are reduced following statin therapy. In patients with MI or CAD and on DAPT, statins significantly lower platelet reactivity in response to various platelet-activating stimuli including AA, collagen, thrombin, and ADP.[31,32] This response is mediated by NO and is evident on platelet function assays perhaps within 72 hours of initiating therapy.[31,32]

Fibrates (eg, fenofibrate, clofibrate, gemfibrozil) reduce triglycerides and increase high-density lipoprotein cholesterol by inhibiting the activity of hydroxyl-methylglutaryl coenzyme A.[33] Fibrates also inhibit platelet aggregation by selectively engaging PPARα.[16] Fenofibrate potentiates the platelet inhibitory effect of simvastatin in human platelets stimulated with ADP. Fenofibrate also delays occlusion time and inhibits ex vivo collagen-induced platelet aggregation, which is mediated by suppression of the TXA2 receptor and COX-1 activity.[16,34] Gemfibrozil, the most potent agent in the fibrate class, can mediate NO-dependent inhibition of platelet aggregation stimulated by ADP and decreases platelet reactivity (ie, reduced ADP-stimulated TXB2 secretion) in patients with hypercholesterolemia.[35,36]

In summary, simultaneous management of dyslipidemia with statins and/or fibrates and thrombosis with antiplatelet therapy is an optimal therapeutic strategy in preventing and treating CVD. In addition to the lipid-lowering effect associated with prevention of CVD, the antihyperlipidemic drugs also affect PPAR pathways to potentiate the antithrombotic effect of DAPT.

Thromboxane Antagonists

Overproduction of TXA2, the main product derived from AA metabolism in platelets, has been linked to multiple thrombotic disorders including MI and atherosclerosis.[37] Although aspirin is an effective and inexpensive therapy for inhibiting TXA2-mediated platelet activation, it is strongly associated with gastrointestinal bleeding and hemorrhagic stroke in patients with comparatively low cardiovascular risk, and there are certain populations that do not respond to aspirin (ie, "aspirin resistance").[38–40] Thus, alternative therapies targeting TXA2 that exhibit a better benefit-to-risk profile would be advantageous.

TXA2 stimulates platelet activity and aggregation by interacting with the TP receptor. The TP receptor is also activated by many extraplatelet sources of TXA2 including the prostaglandins (PGs), PG endoperoxides, and isoprostanes.[41] These extraplatelet sources of TXA2 are less sensitive to aspirin therapy, especially when only a low dose of aspirin is administered once daily.[41] Furthermore, monocytes and macrophages of the immune system produce TXA2 via the COX-2 pathway, which has a higher threshold of inhibition by aspirin than COX-1. TXA2-mediated platelet activation is inhibited either through direct blockade of the platelet surface TP receptor or by inhibition of the enzyme thromboxane synthase (TXS) (see **Fig. 1**).

TP receptor antagonists (eg, terutroban, sulotroban, ifetroban, GR 32191, SQ 29548) inhibit the TXA2 pathway by blocking the downstream signaling mediators of TXA2 receptors. TP receptor antagonists could be more desirable than aspirin in reducing cardiovascular risk because they block all TP receptor agonists, whereas aspirin has no effect on isoprostanes and endoperoxides, which are produced through mechanisms other than COX-1.[42] This promiscuous, nonselective blockade of TP receptors by TP antagonists may explain why aspirin has limited benefits in patients with type 2 diabetes, who exhibit elevated urinary TXA2 metabolites and platelet "hyperreactivity" caused by oxidative stress-induced generation of isoprostanes.[43] Moreover, TP receptor antagonism spares COX-1, COX-2, or any prostanoid synthesis pathway, thereby preserving the cardioprotective vasodilatory effect of prostacyclin (PGI2).[41] Although promising in theory, TP receptor antagonists have not been extremely efficacious in clinical trials, particularly the PERFORM trial, where terutroban failed to demonstrate superiority over aspirin in secondary prevention of CVD events.[41]

Nevertheless, several of these compounds reduce CVD risk in patient and animal studies, the results of which may pave the way for improved clinical studies in the future.

TXA2 is a platelet activator and potent vasoconstrictor and is formed by the enzymatic conversion of PGH2 to TXA2 by TXS.[41,44] By reducing TXA2 synthesis in platelets, the TXS inhibitors (eg, dazoxiben, dazmagrel, pirmagrel, ozagrel, furegrelate) could be particularly advantageous in TXA2-mediated pathologies, such as thrombosis. As an added benefit, TXS inhibitors increase the production of prostacyclin (PGI$_2$), which prevents platelet aggregation and vasodilates. The orally active dazoxiben has been the most commonly used TXS inhibitor clinically. More efficacious compounds that successfully target TXS and the TP receptor with a synergistic effect are currently in development.[45]

Considering their straightforward mechanisms of actions, the identification and characterization of TXS inhibitors and TP receptor antagonists ushered the advent of new and improved antiplatelet therapy for reducing CVD risk.[46] Having been regarded as being too similar to aspirin and not nearly as cost-effective, however, they were essentially abandoned by the pharmaceutical industry.[42] Although TXS inhibitors display the beneficial effects of reducing TXA2 synthesis and enhancing the generation of prostacyclin through the production of endoperoxides, these same endoperoxides can have the deleterious effect of inadvertently triggering platelet activation. Renewed efforts have been directed toward the development of a single compound that possesses the activities of both drug classes, and ongoing research indicates that such a dual inhibitor may be more powerful than either aspirin or drugs with the single actions.[41]

Indeed, dual TP receptor and TXS inhibitors (eg, DT-TX 30) have shown promise in reducing CVD risk in human and animal studies. They circumvent the problematic effect of endoperoxides because of TXS inhibition by blocking the TP receptor.[47] In type 1 diabetic rats, DT-TX 30 inhibits TXS and increases prostacyclin production with more potency than dazoxiben.[48] BM-567, a chemical derivative of the diuretic torsemide, is a novel thromboxane modulator that blocks TP receptors and prevents AA-, collagen-, and ADP-stimulated platelet aggregation.[49] BM-573, another dual TXS inhibitor and TP receptor antagonist, prevents MI in rats and similar observations have been made with BM-531 in human platelets.[50,51]

PREDICTING AND PREVENTING BLEEDING

Bleeding is the most notable risk of antiplatelet therapy during PCI and can increase health care costs, length of hospital stay, and mortality. Estimates of rates of periprocedure or post-procedure bleeding range from 1.7% to 5.8%, with half of the events occurring at the PCI access site and the remaining half from other locations, primarily gastrointestinal.[52] Approximately 12% of deaths after PCI are attributed to periprocedure or post-procedure major bleeding.[53] Critical care nurses are poised to assist with identification of patients at high risk of PCI-associated bleeding and to recommend evidence-based bleeding-avoidance strategies to reduce costs and improve patient outcomes.

The risk factors most strongly associated with PCI-related bleeding include older age (>65 years), female gender, body mass index at extremes (either overweight or underweight), acute presentation (shock, ST-segment elevation MI, Killip class >2 at admission), medical comorbidities (renal failure, anemia, history of bleeding), increased white blood cells, or decreased hemoglobin.[54,55] Point-based models have been developed to assist with prediction of bleeding risk based on these clinical and laboratory values.[54,55] The system developed by Mehran and colleagues[55] factors in six baseline measures plus the procedural anticoagulation regimen to assign patients into a low, moderate, high, or very high risk score (**Table 2**). If a patient is determined to have a significant risk of PCI-related bleeding using one of the scoring systems mentioned previously, then critical care nurses should discuss the use of bleeding-avoidance strategies with the interprofessional health care team.[52,56] Hospitals that have widely implemented evidence-based bleeding-avoidance strategies have reduced bleeding rates compared with hospitals with low use of these strategies.[57]

The ACUITY trial demonstrated a 50% reduction in PCI-related bleeding when bivalirudin was used in place of GP inhibitors as the preferred antithrombotic agent.[58] However, bivalirudin is associated with a higher acquisition cost than most GP inhibitors. Use of the radial artery as the PCI access site decreases bleeding complications compared with femoral access (1.2% vs 3% incidence of hematoma at the access site, respectively).[59] Limitations of this strategy include artery occlusion and catheter entrapment; however, future improvements to device design could reduce these risks. When radial artery access fails, femoral access is required, leaving patients with multiple puncture sites that are prone to hematoma. Finally, vascular closure devices may offer improved hemostasis compared with manual compression of the femoral access site, but they also carry a risk of infection or leg ischemia if improperly deployed.[56]

REVERSAL AGENTS

Life-threatening bleeding is a serious complication that is associated with antiplatelet therapy. Even when bleeding is not considered life-threatening, it may be associated with an increased risk of recurrent ischemic events and death.[60] Consequently, reversing the effects of an antiplatelet drug may be required. Although there are no $P2Y_{12}$-specific reversal agents, some possible strategies for reversal of antiplatelets and aspirin in the setting of life-threatening bleeding include desmopressin and platelet transfusions.[61]

Bleeding caused by aspirin is partially reversed within 15 to 30 minutes by infusion of either a platelet concentrate or desmopressin (1-deamino-8-D-arginine vasopressin).[61] Bleeding associated with prasugrel or clopidogrel treatment is resolved using similar strategies. The desmopressin infusion should be dosed at 0.3 to 0.4 µg/kg in 100 mL of normal saline over 30 minutes.[61] However, desmopressin is contraindicated in patients with a creatinine clearance less than 50 mL/min and in patients with hyponatremia or a history of hyponatremia. Most importantly, desmopressin increases serum levels of von Willebrand factor and other proaggregating clotting factors and is, thus, contraindicated in patients with CVD because of the high risk of thrombosis.[62,63] Current guidelines recommend using two to three units of platelets to reverse the antiplatelet effect of $P2Y_{12}$ inhibitors or aspirin.[62]

A potential antidote for the reversal of ticagrelor is albumin. Because ticagrelor is a reversible inhibitor of the $P2Y_{12}$ receptor and is highly bound to protein (>99%), the fraction of drug not bound to the platelet $P2Y_{12}$ receptor is generally bound to albumin and other plasma carrier proteins.[64] Platelet transfusions have not yielded favorable results when treating bleeds associated with ticagrelor. This observation is likely because plasma ticagrelor can easily transfer to the donor platelets.[65] However, in vitro studies indicate that albumin or human plasma can be administered to bind the excess ticagrelor, thereby reducing the potential for antiplatelet activity.[66,67] A larger clinical trial is needed to help quantify any in vivo effects and to establish proper dosing regimens.

Table 2
Integer-based risk score for non-CABG-related major bleeding within 30 days of patient presentation with ACS

Factor							Add to Score
Gender	Male			Female			
	0			+8			
Age (y)	<50	50-59	60-69	70-79	≥80		
	0	+3	+6	+9	+12		
Serum creatinine (mg/dL)	<1.0	1.0-	1.2-	1.4-	1.6-	1.8-	≥2.0
	0	+2	+3	+5	+6	+8	+10
White blood cell count (giga/L)	<10	10-	12-	14-	16-	18-	≥20
	0	+2	+3	+5	+6	+8	+10
Anemia	No			Yes			
	0			+6			
Presentation	STEMI		NSTEMI – Raised biomarkers		NSTEMI – Normal biomarkers		
	+6		+2		0		
Antithrombotic medications	Heparin plus a glycoprotein inhibitor			Bivalirudin monotherapy			
	0			−5			

Total score[a]	0	5	10	15	20	25	30	35	40
Risk of bleeding (%)	0.9	1.6	2.8	4.7	7.9	12.9	20.4	30.7	43.5

As described by Mehran and colleagues,[55] factors including gender, age, serum creatinine, white blood cell count, presence or absence of anemia, presentation with or without STEMI, and raised biomarkers and antithrombotic medication are all used to calculate a total score that translates into a percent risk of bleeding.

Abbreviations: CABG, coronary artery bypass graft; NSTEMI, non-ST-segment elevation myocardial infarction; STEMI, ST-segment elevation myocardial infarction.

From Mehran R, Pocock SJ, Nikolsky E, et al. A risk score to predict bleeding in patients with acute coronary syndromes. J Am Coll Cardiol 2010;55(23):2560; with permission.

Additionally, MEDI2452 is an investigational monoclonal antibody that is designed to rapidly reverse the bleeding effects of ticagrelor.[68] Currently in development, MEDI2452 functions as an antidote by binding to ticagrelor and its active metabolite, AR-C124910XX. Although MEDI2452 has only been tested in animal models, the results are encouraging. Specifically, ADP-induced platelet aggregation returns to close-to-normal values within 1 hour following its infusion, with no difference in mortality between treated and untreated animals.[68] Phase I human trials are set to begin in 2018. Similar to monoclonal antibody–based antidotes for anticoagulant agents, this drug will initially likely have a high acquisition cost and be reserved for life-threatening bleeding events.

PERSONALIZED ANTIPLATELET THERAPY

The concept of personalized medicine, also known as precision medicine, is still in its infancy and is gradually emerging in clinical practice. In personalized or precision medicine, pharmacotherapy is selected based on an individual's genetics, and the class of $P2Y_{12}$ inhibitors stands out as a strong candidate for this scientific approach.

The $P2Y_{12}$ receptor plays a central role in the development of thrombotic CVD, but its sensitivity is highly variable across patient populations. Genetic variations in the $P2Y_{12}$ receptor have been linked to an increased risk of and susceptibility to CAD.[69] $P2Y_{12}$ receptor activation involves intracellular signaling that is mediated by the G protein subunit beta 3 (GNB3) and the platelet endothelial aggregation receptor-1 (PEAR1). Genetic variations in the $P2Y_{12}$ receptor, PEAR1 and GNB3 have all been linked to an impaired antiplatelet response to $P2Y_{12}$ receptor antagonists.[70,71]

Additionally, patients with certain genetic variations (ie, polymorphisms) may metabolize drugs at rates that are different from those of the general population, leading to altered pharmacokinetics and potential differences in CVD outcomes. Crucial to the metabolism of drugs, cytochrome P-450 (CYP) enzymes metabolize potentially toxic compounds including drugs, primarily in the liver. CYP family 2 subfamily C member 19 (CYP2C19) has been an area of extensive research for antiplatelet therapy because of its role in the metabolic conversion of clopidogrel, an inactive precursor molecule, to its active metabolite. Reduced function of CYP2C19, due to gene mutations, would manifest as low serum levels of bioactive clopidogrel, leading to lack of platelet inhibition, high platelet reactivity, and increased thrombotic risk.[72] The FDA labeling for clopidogrel warns that patients who are CYP2C19 poor metabolizers may have diminished effectiveness of a drug as compared with patients with normal CYP2C19 function.[73] Moreover, genetic polymorphisms in CYP3A (specifically CYP3A4*1G and CYP3A5*3), which cause loss in the function of the enzyme, does not significantly influence pharmacokinetics of ticagrelor, but it does significantly influence the pharmacokinetics of the main active metabolite of ticagrelor. Increased exposure to the active metabolite has not been shown to increase bleeding risk, however.[74]

Polymorphic genes encoding drug transporter proteins may also result in interindividual variations in the pharmacokinetics of drugs. Some $P2Y_{12}$ inhibitors use efflux and/or influx drug transporter proteins to cross biologic membranes.[75] Clopidogrel is a substrate to the efflux transporter protein ATP-binding cassette subfamily B member 1 (ABCB1). Conflicting reports exist on the impact of an ABCB1 C3435T polymorphism on the pharmacokinetics of clopidogrel, with some studies associating the gene variant with decreased plasma clopidogrel concentrations and decreased platelet inhibition, and others showing no effect.[71,75]

Consequently, an equivalent dose of a drug administered to one patient may not result in comparable pharmacokinetic outcomes in other patients. This interpatient variability in response could, therefore, require that a dosage adjustment be performed based on each patient's genetic makeup. The future of antiplatelet therapy could entail the personalization of medication regimens by cardiologists, guided by pharmacogenomic and platelet function testing (PFT), to maximize clinical outcomes and minimize adverse events. However, multiple major clinical trials have failed to demonstrate that tailored antiplatelet therapy can improve clinical outcomes.[72,76–79] It is unclear whether these negative results are caused by a lack of efficacy or limitations in the study designs, namely a low event rate of the primary efficacy outcome.

Despite a lack of evidence of improved clinical outcomes, published guidelines can help to direct clinicians in determining when to order PFT and pharmacogenomic testing and how to apply the results to patient care.[4,73] In particular, PFT may be useful in clopidogrel-treated patients with ACS and a history of stent thrombosis.[4] If PFT results fall to less than the targeted therapeutic range, then the patient has low platelet reactivity and an increased risk of bleeding. Conversely, PFT results higher than therapeutic values indicate high platelet reactivity and increased thrombotic or ischemic risk. Genetic testing for CYP2C19 loss-of-function alleles should be considered on a case-by-case basis, especially for patients who experience recurrent ACS events despite ongoing therapy with clopidogrel.[73] As usage of pharmacogenomics and PFT increases, critical care nurses will be integral members of the multidisciplinary care team in terms of modifying antiplatelet therapy to optimize patient care outcomes.[4,80]

DRUG INTERACTIONS

The large number of comorbidities associated with CVD (eg, diabetes, hypertension, hyperlipidemia, obesity) often implies polypharmacy and complicates antiplatelet therapy selection by introducing drug interactions that alter the expected pharmacokinetics and pharmacodynamics of established medication regimens. The widely used $P2Y_{12}$ inhibitor clopidogrel is a prodrug that must be metabolized to its active metabolite by CYP450 2C19, a metabolic pathway shared by many other common medications including proton-pump inhibitors (particularly omeprazole) and certain lipophilic statins (eg, atorvastatin, simvastatin, lovastatin). The potential for increased incidence of cardiovascular events in patients taking clopidogrel and one of these other agents has been examined in *in vitro* studies, retrospective observational trials, and prospective randomized trials with mixed results and no definitive conclusions. It seems certain that clopidogrel cotherapy with either statins or proton-pump inhibitors can negatively impact serum clopidogrel concentrations and decrease the antiplatelet effect as measured by PFT.[81–83] Whether this decrease in drug exposure results in increased harm as measured by increased cardiovascular events is less clear, and most studies have shown no increase in CVD events.[84,85]

A second drug interaction of particular interest to the critical care nurse is the interaction displayed between the $P2Y_{12}$ inhibitors and morphine.[86] Because of the seizing effect of opioids on the gut, decreased gut motility and decreased absorption of orally administered antiplatelet agents leads to a delay in the therapeutic antiplatelet effect ranging between 2 and 6 hours.[86] Morphine stalls the antiplatelet effect of the $P2Y_{12}$ inhibitors and can result in a statistically and clinically significant increase in mortality.[86] Similarly, fentanyl slows gastric emptying and inhibits the antiplatelet effect of ticagrelor by more than 4 hours.[87] Despite the potentially significant impact of these findings, it is not currently recommended to withhold opioid medications from patients suffering with pain until a larger trial has been conducted.[86,87]

SUMMARY

Critical care nurses are often charged with administering antiplatelet medications for patients suffering from CVD and related sequalae. It is, therefore, imperative that nursing personnel understand how these drugs work and be aware of the risks associated with each of them. Moreover, nursing staff should maintain a heightened awareness for situations where the risk of bleeding may be elevated. Specifically, they should be able to identify those patients who, because of genetic factors or comorbidities, could be prone to higher incidences of bleeding. Furthermore, they should recognize the strategies that are available for avoiding or reversing bleeds and possess an appreciation for how personalized antiplatelet therapy could improve patient outcomes. Moreover, nursing staff should understand that critical drug interactions may either enhance or delay the antiplatelet effect of P2Y$_{12}$ inhibitors to influence patient outcomes. Taken altogether, as more subtleties are discovered about various antiplatelet drug classes, the therapeutic regimen will become increasingly patient- and disease-specific and tailored based on genetics, comorbidities, and drug interaction potential, with the ultimate goal of reducing CVD risk.

REFERENCES

1. Benjamin EJ, Blaha MJ, Chiuve SE, et al. Heart disease and stroke statistics–2017 update: a report from the American Heart Association. Circulation 2017. https://doi.org/10.1161/CIR.0000000000000485.
2. American Heart Association. Cardiovascular disease: a costly burden for America. Projections through 2035. Am Hear Assoc 2017;7. doi:1/17DS11775.
3. Behan MWH, Storey RF. Antiplatelet therapy in cardiovascular disease. Postgrad Med J 2004;80(941):155–64.
4. Tantry US, Bonello L, Aradi D, et al. Consensus and update on the definition of on-treatment platelet reactivity to adenosine diphosphate associated with ischemia and bleeding. J Am Coll Cardiol 2013;62(24):2261–73.
5. O'connor CT, Kiernan TJ, Yan BP. The genetic basis of antiplatelet and anticoagulant therapy: a pharmacogenetic review of newer antiplatelets (clopidogrel, prasugrel and ticagrelor) and anticoagulants (dabigatran, rivaroxaban, apixaban and edoxaban). Expert Opin Drug Metab Toxicol 2017;13(7):725–39.
6. Moon JY, Franchi F, Rollini F, et al. Role of genetic testing in patients undergoing percutaneous coronary intervention. Expert Rev Clin Pharmacol 2018;11(2):151–64.
7. Hochholzer W, Ruff CT, Mesa RA, et al. Variability of individual platelet reactivity over time in patients treated with clopidogrel: insights from the ELEVATE-TIMI 56 trial. J Am Coll Cardiol 2014;64(4):361–8.
8. Freynhofer MK, Bruno V, Brozovic I, et al. Variability of on-treatment platelet reactivity in patients on clopidogrel. Platelets 2014;25(5):328–36.
9. Linden MD, Tran H, Woods R, et al. High platelet reactivity and antiplatelet therapy resistance. Semin Thromb Hemost 2012;38(2):200–12.
10. Wallentin L. P2Y(12) inhibitors: differences in properties and mechanisms of action and potential consequences for clinical use. Eur Heart J 2009;30(16):1964–77.
11. Baker DE, Ingram KT. Cangrelor. Hosp Pharm 2015;50(10):922–9.
12. Bhatt DL, Lincoff AM, Gibson CM, et al. Intravenous platelet blockade with cangrelor during PCI. N Engl J Med 2009;361(24):2330–41.
13. Waite LH, Phan YL, Spinler SA. Cangrelor: a novel intravenous antiplatelet agent with a questionable future. Pharmacotherapy 2014;34(10):1061–76.

14. Angiolillo DJ, Rollini F, Storey RF, et al. International expert consensus on switch-ing platelet P2Y12 receptor-inhibiting therapies. Circulation 2017;136(20): 1955–75.
15. Pahan K. Lipid-lowering drugs. Cell Mol Life Sci 2006;63(10):1165–78.
16. Ali FY, Armstrong PCJ, Dhanji ARA, et al. Antiplatelet actions of statins and fi-brates are mediated by PPARs. Arterioscler Thromb Vasc Biol 2009;29(5): 706–11.
17. Min L, Shao S, Wu X, et al. Anti-inflammatory and anti-thrombogenic effects of atorvastatin in acute ischemic stroke. Neural Regen Res 2013;8(23):2144–54.
18. Gaddam V, Li DY, Mehta JL. Anti-thrombotic effects of atorvastatin: an effect un-related to lipid lowering. J Cardiovasc Pharmacol Ther 2002;7(4):247–53.
19. Puccetti L, Pasqui AL, Auteri A, et al. Mechanisms for antiplatelet action of statins. Curr Drug Targets Cardiovasc Haematol Disord 2005;5(2):121–6.
20. Varga T, Czimmerer Z, Nagy L. PPARs are a unique set of fatty acid regulated transcription factors controlling both lipid metabolism and inflammation. Biochim Biophys Acta 2011;1812(8):1007–22.
21. Du H, Hu H, Zheng H, et al. Effects of peroxisome proliferator-activated receptor γ in simvastatin antiplatelet activity: influences on cAMP and mitogen-activated protein kinases. Thromb Res 2014;134(1):111–20.
22. Morrow JD, Minton TA, Mukundan CR, et al. Free radical-induced generation of isoprostanes in vivo. Evidence for the formation of D-ring and E-ring isopros-tanes. J Biol Chem 1994;269(6):4317–26.
23. Liu T, Stern A, Roberts LJ, et al. The isoprostanes: novel prostaglandin-like prod-ucts of the free radical-catalyzed peroxidation of arachidonic acid. J Biomed Sci 1999;6(4):226–35.
24. Mendelsohn ME, O'Neill S, George D, et al. Inhibition of fibrinogen binding to human platelets by S-nitroso-N-acetylcysteine. J Biol Chem 1990;265(31): 19028–34.
25. Lowenstein CJ, Dinerman JL, Snyder SH. Nitric oxide: a physiologic messenger. Ann Intern Med 1994;120(3):227–37.
26. Wang GR, Zhu Y, Halushka PV, et al. Mechanism of platelet inhibition by nitric ox-ide: in vivo phosphorylation of thromboxane receptor by cyclic GMP-dependent protein kinase. Proc Natl Acad Sci U S A 1998;95(9):4888–93.
27. Violi F, Carnevale R, Pastori D, et al. Antioxidant and antiplatelet effects of ator-vastatin by Nox2 inhibition. Trends Cardiovasc Med 2014;24(4):142–8.
28. Pignatelli P, Carnevale R, Pastori D, et al. Immediate antioxidant and antiplatelet effect of atorvastatin via inhibition of Nox2. Circulation 2012;126(1):92–103.
29. Badimon L, Suades R, Fuentes E, et al. Role of platelet-derived microvesicles as crosstalk mediators in atherothrombosis and future pharmacology targets: a link between inflammation, atherosclerosis, and thrombosis. Front Pharmacol 2016;7: 293.
30. Wang ZT, Wang Z, Hu YW. Possible roles of platelet-derived microparticles in atherosclerosis. Atherosclerosis 2016;248:10–6.
31. Matetzky S, Fefer P, Shenkman B, et al. Statins have an early antiplatelet effect in patients with acute myocardial infarction. Platelets 2011;22(2):103–10.
32. Verdoia M, Pergolini P, Rolla R, et al. Impact of high-dose statins on vitamin D levels and platelet function in patients with coronary artery disease. Thromb Res 2017;150:90–5.
33. Feingold K, Grunfeld C. Triglyceride lowering drugs. Endotext 2000;1–52.
34. Lee JJ, Jin YR, Yu JY, et al. Antithrombotic and antiplatelet activities of fenofi-brate, a lipid-lowering drug. Atherosclerosis 2009;206(2):375–82.

35. Laustiola K, Lassila R, Koskinen P, et al. Gemfibrozil decreases platelet reactivity in patients with hypercholesterolemia during physical stress. Clin Pharmacol Ther 1988;43(3):302–7.
36. Sharina IG, Sobolevsky M, Papakyriakou A, et al. The fibrate gemfibrozil is a NO- and haem-independent activator of soluble guanylyl cyclase: in vitro studies. Br J Pharmacol 2015;172(9):2316–29.
37. Smyth EM. Thromboxane and the thromboxane receptor in cardiovascular disease. Clin Lipidol 2010;5(2):209–19.
38. Huang ES, Strate LL, Ho WW, et al. Long-term use of aspirin and the risk of gastrointestinal bleeding. Am J Med 2011;124(5):426–33.
39. Gorelick PB, Weisman SM. Risk of hemorrhagic stroke with aspirin use: an update. Stroke 2005;36(8):1801–7.
40. Wong S, Appleberg M, Ward CM, et al. Aspirin resistance in cardiovascular disease: a review. Eur J Vasc Endovasc Surg 2004;27(5):456–65.
41. Davì G, Santilli F, Vazzana N. Thromboxane receptors antagonists and/or synthase inhibitors. Handb Exp Pharmacol 2012;210:261–86.
42. Ritter JM. TP receptor antagonists (TXRAs): expensive irrelevance or wonder drugs strangled at birth? Br J Clin Pharmacol 2011;71(6):801–3.
43. Cangemi R, Pignatelli P, Carnevale R, et al. Platelet isoprostane overproduction in diabetic patients treated with aspirin. Diabetes 2012;61(6):1626–32.
44. Paul BZS, Jin J, Kunapuli SP. Molecular mechanism of thromboxane A2-induced platelet aggregation. J Biol Chem 1999;274(41):29108–14.
45. Krishna A, Yadav A. Lead compound design for TPR/COX dual inhibition. J Mol Model 2012;18(9):4397–408.
46. Vermylen J, Deckmyn H. Thromboxane synthase inhibitors and receptor antagonists. Cardiovasc Drugs Ther 1992;6(1):29–33.
47. De La Cruz JP, Villalobos MA, Escalante R, et al. Effects of the selective inhibition of platelet thromboxane synthesis on the platelet-subendothelium interaction. Br J Pharmacol 2002;137(7):1082–8.
48. De La Cruz JP, Moreno A, Ruiz-Ruiz MI, et al. Effect of DT-TX 30, a combined thromboxane synthase inhibitor and thromboxane receptor antagonist, on retinal vascularity in experimental diabetes mellitus. Thromb Res 2000;97(3):125–31.
49. Dogné JM, De Leval X, Kolh P, et al. Pharmacological evaluation of the novel thromboxane modulator BM-567 (I/II). Effects of BM-567 on platelet function. Prostaglandins Leukot Essent Fatty Acids 2003;68(1):49–54.
50. Dogne JM, Rolin S, de Leval X, et al. Pharmacology of the thromboxane receptor antagonist and thromboxane synthase inhibitor BM-531. Cardiovasc Drug Rev 2001;19(2):87–96.
51. Rolin S, Petein M, Tchana-Sato V, et al. BM-573, a dual thromboxane synthase inhibitor and thromboxane receptor antagonist, prevents pig myocardial infarction induced by coronary thrombosis. J Pharmacol Exp Ther 2003;1:59–306.
52. Shuvy M, Ko DT. Bleeding after percutaneous coronary intervention: can we still ignore the obvious? Open Heart 2014;1(1):e000036.
53. Kwok CS, Ao SV, Myint PK, et al. Major bleeding after percutaneous coronary intervention and risk of subsequent mortality: a systematic review and meta-analysis. Open Heart 2014;1(1):e000021.
54. Rao SV, McCoy LA, Spertus JA, et al. An updated bleeding model to predict the risk of post-procedure bleeding among patients undergoing percutaneous coronary intervention. JACC Cardiovasc Interv 2013;6(9):897–904.
55. Mehran R, Pocock SJ, Nikolsky E, et al. A risk score to predict bleeding in patients with acute coronary syndromes. J Am Coll Cardiol 2010;55(23):2556–66.

56. Bates ER. Bleeding avoidance strategies, performance measures, and the emperor's new clothes. JACC Cardiovasc Interv 2016;9(8):780–3.
57. Vora AN, Peterson ED, McCoy LA, et al. The impact of bleeding avoidance strategies on hospital-level variation in bleeding rates following percutaneous coronary intervention insights from the national cardiovascular data registry CathPCI registry. JACC Cardiovasc Interv 2016;9(8):771–9.
58. Stone GW, McLaurin BT, Cox DA, et al. Bivalirudin for patients with acute coronary syndromes. N Engl J Med 2006;355(21):2203–16.
59. Jolly SS, Yusuf S, Cairns J, et al. Radial versus femoral access for coronary angiography and intervention in patients with acute coronary syndromes (RIVAL): a randomised, parallel group, multicentre trial. Lancet 2011;377(9775):1409–20.
60. Eikelboom JW, Mehta SR, Anand SS. Adverse impact of bleeding on prognosis in patients with acute coronary syndromes. Circulation 2006;114(8):774–82.
61. Levi MM, Eerenberg E, Löwenberg E, et al. Bleeding in patients using new anticoagulants or antiplatelet agents: risk factors and management. Neth J Med 2010;68(2):68–76.
62. Makris M, Van Veen JJ, Tait CR, et al. Guideline on the management of bleeding in patients on antithrombotic agents. Br J Haematol 2013;160(1):35–46.
63. Levine M, Swenson S, McCormick T, et al. Reversal of thienopyridine-induced platelet dysfunction following desmopressin administration. J Med Toxicol 2013;9(2):139–43.
64. Sillén H, Cook M, Davis P. Determination of unbound ticagrelor and its active metabolite (AR-C124910XX) in human plasma by equilibrium dialysis and LC-MS/MS. J Chromatogr B Analyt Technol Biomed Life Sci 2011;879(23): 2315–22.
65. Teng R, Carlson GF, Nylander S, et al. Effects of autologous platelet transfusion on platelet inhibition in ticagrelor- and clopidogrel-treated subjects. J Thromb Haemost 2016. https://doi.org/10.1111/jth.13511.
66. Schoener L, Jellinghaus S, Richter B, et al. Reversal of the platelet inhibitory effect of the P2Y12inhibitors clopidogrel, prasugrel, and ticagrelor in vitro: a new approach to an old issue. Clin Res Cardiol 2017;106(11):868–74.
67. Bertling A, Fender AC, Schüngel L, et al. Reversibility of platelet P2Y12 inhibition by platelet supplementation: ex vivo and in vitro comparisons of prasugrel, clopidogrel and ticagrelor. J Thromb Haemost 2018;16(6):1089–98.
68. Pehrsson S, Johansson KJ, Janefeldt A, et al. Hemostatic effects of the ticagrelor antidote MEDI2452 in pigs treated with ticagrelor on a background of aspirin. J Thromb Haemost 2017;15(6):1213–22.
69. Yang HH, Chen Y, Gao CY. Associations of P2Y12R gene polymorphisms with susceptibility to coronary heart disease and clinical efficacy of antiplatelet treatment with clopidogrel. Cardiovasc Ther 2016;34(6):460–7.
70. Li MP, Tang J, Wen ZP, et al. Influence of P2Y12 polymorphisms on platelet activity but not ex-vivo antiplatelet effect of ticagrelor in healthy Chinese male subjects. Blood Coagul Fibrinolysis 2015;26(8):874–81.
71. Sridharan K, Kataria R, Tolani D, et al. Evaluation of CYP2C19, P2Y12, and ABCB1 polymorphisms and phenotypic response to clopidogrel in healthy Indian adults. Indian J Pharmacol 2016;48(4):350.
72. Xi Z, Fang F, Wang J, et al. CYP2C19 genotype and adverse cardiovascular outcomes after stent implantation in clopidogrel-treated Asian populations: a systematic review and meta-analysis. Platelets 2017;1–12. https://doi.org/10.1080/09537104.2017.1413178.

73. Jneid H. The 2012 ACCF/AHA focused update of the unstable angina/non-ST-elevation myocardial infarction (UA/NSTEMI) guideline: a critical appraisal. Methodist Debakey Cardiovasc J 2012;8(3):26–30.
74. Liu S, Shi X, Tian X, et al. Effect of CYP3A4*1G and CYP3A5*3 polymorphisms on pharmacokinetics and pharmacodynamics of ticagrelor in healthy Chinese subjects. Front Pharmacol 2017;8:176.
75. Wang XQ, Shen CL, Wang BN, et al. Genetic polymorphisms of CYP2C19*2 and ABCB1 C3435T affect the pharmacokinetic and pharmacodynamic responses to clopidogrel in 401 patients with acute coronary syndrome. Gene 2015;558(2): 200–7.
76. Price MJ, Berger PB, Teirstein PS, et al. Standard- vs high-dose clopidogrel based on platelet function testing after percutaneous coronary intervention: the GRAVITAS randomized trial. JAMA 2011;305(11):1097–105.
77. Trenk D, Stone GW, Gawaz M, et al. A randomized trial of prasugrel versus clopidogrel in patients with high platelet reactivity on clopidogrel after elective percutaneous coronary intervention with implantation of drug-eluting stents: results of the TRIGGER-PCI (testing platelet reactivity. J Am Coll Cardiol 2012; 59(24):2159–64.
78. Collet J-P, Cuisset T, Rangé G, et al. Bedside monitoring to adjust antiplatelet therapy for coronary stenting. N Engl J Med 2012;367(22):2100–9.
79. Cayla G, Cuisset T, Silvain J, et al. Platelet function monitoring to adjust antiplatelet therapy in elderly patients stented for an acute coronary syndrome (ANTARCTIC): an open-label, blinded-endpoint, randomised controlled superiority trial. Lancet 2016;388(10055):2015–22.
80. Price MJ. Bedside evaluation of thienopyridine antiplatelet therapy. Circulation 2009;119(19):2625–32.
81. Lau WC, Waskell LA, Watkins PB, et al. Atorvastatin reduces the ability of clopidogrel to inhibit platelet aggregation: a new drug-drug interaction. Circulation 2003;107(1):32–7.
82. Neubauer H, Günesdogan B, Hanefeld C, et al. Lipophilic statins interfere with the inhibitory effects of clopidogrel on platelet function: a flow cytometry study. Eur Heart J 2003;24(19):1744–9.
83. Frelinger AL, Lee RD, Mulford DJ, et al. A randomized, 2-period, crossover design study to assess the effects of dexlansoprazole, lansoprazole, esomeprazole, and omeprazole on the steady-state pharmacokinetics and pharmacodynamics of clopidogrel in healthy volunteers. J Am Coll Cardiol 2012;59(14): 1304–11.
84. Zhang JR, Wang DQ, Du J, et al. Efficacy of clopidogrel and clinical outcome when clopidogrel is coadministered with atorvastatin and lansoprazole: a prospective, randomized, controlled trial. Medicine (Baltimore) 2015;94(50):e2262.
85. Bouziana SD. Clinical relevance of clopidogrel-proton pump inhibitors interaction. World J Gastrointest Pharmacol Ther 2015;6(2):17.
86. Kubica J, Kubica A, Jilma B, et al. Impact of morphine on antiplatelet effects of oral P2Y12 receptor inhibitors. Int J Cardiol 2016;215:201–8.
87. McEvoy JW, Ibrahim K, Kickler TS, et al. Effect of intravenous fentanyl on ticagrelor absorption and platelet inhibition among patients undergoing percutaneous coronary intervention: the PACIFY randomized clinical trial (platelet aggregation with ticagrelor inhibition and fentanyl). Circulation 2018;137(3):307–9.
88. Dobesh PP, Oestreich JH. Ticagrelor: pharmacokinetics, pharmacodynamics, clinical efficacy, and safety. Pharmacotherapy 2014;34(10):1077–90.

Comprehensive Nursing Management for Valvular Disease

Susan Lee, RN, APRN, FNP-BC

KEYWORDS

- Nursing management • Mitral stenosis • Mitral regurgitation • Aortic stenosis
- Aortic regurgitation

KEY POINTS

- Accurate assessment and early diagnosis of valvular heart disease facilitates optimal treatment.
- Aortic stenosis is treated pharmaceutically until the pressure gradient exceeds 40 mm HG requiring surgical treatment.
- In the absence of contraindications beta-blockers are effective in management of mitral stenosis.
- Client education focuses on progressive exercise, medications, and symptoms that warrant provider notification.

ASSESSMENT

If valvular heart disease is suspected, the physical assessment should focus on dysfunctional manifestations.[1,2] A client may have a murmur, dysrhythmia, or symptoms of heart failure. Depending on the degree of failure, findings may include dyspnea, orthopnea, crackles, cough, decreased blood pressure, nausea, vomiting, ascites, dependent edema, jugular venous distension, S3 gallop, enlarged spleen and liver, decreased urine output, fatigue, confusion, or anxiety (**Table 1**).

Routine serial surveillance will include chest radiograph to evaluate heart size and pulmonary status and transesophageal echocardiography (TEE) to evaluate valve function and pumping capacity. Other case-specific testing may include a cardiac stress test, computed tomography (CT), or cardiac catheterization to determine compromised cardiac status, function, and eligibility for applicable treatment interventions.[3]

The author has nothing to disclose.
School of Nursing, Louisiana State University Health, 1900 Gravier Street, Room 328, New Orleans, LA 70112, USA
E-mail address: slee17@lsuhsc.edu

Crit Care Nurs Clin N Am 31 (2019) 31–38
https://doi.org/10.1016/j.cnc.2018.11.002
0899-5885/19/Published by Elsevier Inc.

Table 1
Assessment findings

	Auscultation	Murmur	EKG	Diagnostic	Pulse Pressure
Mital valve prolapse	Midsystolic click at apex S3	Late systolic	Normal T-wave inversion ST depression VTACH PVC Atrial fibrillation	Echocardiogram 2-dimensional and Doppler	
Aortic stenosis	Decreased intensity S2 S4	Mid-late systolic May radiate to carotids		Echocardiogram	Narrowed
Aortic regurgitation		Diastolic	Sinus tachycardia	Echocardiogram CT	Widened
Mitral stenosis	Opening snap after S2	Apical diastolic	Atrial fibrillation Palpitations	TEE	

Abbreviations: CT, computed tomography; EKG, electrocardiogram; PVC, premature ventricular contraction; S2, second heart sound; S3, third heart sound; S4, fourth heart sound; TEE, transesophageal echocardiography.

CLASSIFICATION

The 2014 AHA/ACC guidelines describe severity criteria classifications stages. Clients with Class "A" classification have risk factors for VHD. Clients with Class "B" have progressive VHD, are asymptomatic, and have mild to moderate severity staging. Clients with Class "C" are termed as asymptomatic severe, with further specification to be either "C1" with ventricular compensation or "C2" with ventricular decompensation. Clients with Class "D" are overtly symptomatic and termed severe.[4]

AORTIC STENOSIS

As the population is aging, the incidence of aortic stenosis is likewise increasing.[5] Normally the aortic valve is a tricuspid formation; however, a congenital bicuspid formation predisposes up to 2% of the population to aortic stenosis. The traditionally occurring manifestation entails the aortic valve becoming sclerotic and calcified altering its patency.[4,5]

Initial suspect assessment findings include a mid-late systolic murmur radiating to the carotids. Although many are asymptomatic, the need for a chest radiograph is to assess heart size and TEE to determine systolic function, cardiac blood flow, and valve function. Further testing may include an exercise stress test, dobutamine stress testing, or cardiac catheterization to establish cardiac function, ejection fraction, and pressure gradient across valves.

Treatment

Since the hypertension is associated with a 2-fold increase in mortality rate compared with those normotensive clients, blood pressure control is paramount. Although diuretics may aid in volume control, they are contraindicated if the cardiac output is compromised by ventricular wall hypertrophy. Conversely, angiotensin-converting enzyme (ACE) inhibitor titration for desired normotensive and added beta-blockers for rate control is most effective.[6]

Aortic valve replacement is recommended for those with symptomatic aortic stenosis or severe aortic stenosis causing a gradient of 40 mm HG or greater. Some interventional cardiologists note that percutaneous balloon aortic dilation may bridge unstable clients until they may tolerate replacement procedures. Both the surgical and the transcatheter aortic valve replacements are associated with risks such as cardiac shock or pulmonary edema.[7,8]

AORTIC REGURGITATION

The overt assessment finding for aortic regurgitation (AR) is chest pain, associated pulmonary edema, and hypotension. Most commonly caused by bicuspid and calcified aortic valve disorder, likely precipitated by trauma or instrumentation, emergent condition requires prompt assessment. Because the TEE is more invasive there are more risks involved, such as esophageal perforation, excessive vasovagal stimulation, and compromised oxygenation. However, it is more sensitive and specific to evaluate the thoracic aorta and the intracardiac structures than the TTE. CT as well is very accurate and able to rapidly assess the range of severity from compromised aortic patency through dissection.[9]

Treatment

For those with chronic AR, there are contradicting findings regarding the use of vasodilators. Recent research studies agree that beta-blockers are contraindicated because the lowered heart rate increases stroke volume, thus increasing the aortic pressure gradient and systolic pressure.

Essentially, there is no conservative measure or pharmaceutical agent indicated to reduce the progression of aortic dilation or dissection. Surgical intervention constituting aortic valve, sinuses, and ascending aorta is necessary in unstable patients or when the aorta diameter is larger than 5.5 cm.[4,10,11]

MITRAL STENOSIS

The staging of mitral stenosis depends on the influence of rheumatic cause, because the progression is gradual after an extended latency period. By contrast, the senile form attributed to calcification of the valve leaflets, worsening stenosis as the left ventricle enlarges. Symptomatology may include nonspecific exertional dyspnea and often atrial fibrillation and the associated manifestations. In severe cases, the client develops pulmonary hypertension.[4,12]

Although TEE evaluation is ideal for detecting thrombi, evaluation of valvular dysfunction, commissurotomy eligibility, and hemodynamic status is often achieved using the less invasive TTE. Such serial monitoring to evaluate the disease progression includes pulmonary artery pressures as well as the valve gradients. Exercise testing or heart catheterization evaluates the degree of valvular response when symptomology severity is not consistent with the less invasive TTE result stratification.[13,14]

Treatment

Beta-blockers to control the heart rate and stabilize atrial fibrillation are effective for management of both the asymptomatic and the progressing stages. Considering the frequent atrial fibrillation as well as indurated calcified valves, anticoagulation therapy is often necessary. Nevertheless, a percentage of such clients will still experience embolic sequelae. As the mitral stenotic client becomes symptomatic, most often percutaneous mitral balloon commissurotomy is performed.[13,15,16]

MITRAL REGURGITATION

An inferior ST segment elevation myocardial infarction may cause rupture of a papillary muscle precipitating acute mitral regurgitation. Otherwise, acute onset in the presence of progressive disease may be attributed to spontaneous chordae rupture. Rapidly diagnosed by TTE, even partial supporting chordal damage warrants emergent valve surgery. Depending on associated hemodynamic stability, systemic vasodilatation may facilitate impaired aortic outflow. Likewise, the use of intraaortic balloon counter-pulsation lowers aortic pressures while supporting systolic pressures that may be additionally affected by vasodilation until stabilized for needed surgical intervention.[9,16]

Chronic asymptomatic clients with mitral disease are monitored sequentially by TTE for left ventricular dysfunction. The progression of valve dysfunction or noted symptomology including dyspnea on exertion, exercise intolerance, and manifestations of left ventricular failure escalate that need for repair or valve replacement. Note that those with a rheumatic cause are more likely to need valve replacement as opposed to a repair.[17]

PATIENT EDUCATION

Distributed information should include the pathophysiology and associated symptomology of valvular heart disease. Discharge information should include the manifestations signifying worsening valve dysfunction such as fluid balance dysfunction, breathlessness, and edema. The nurse will review with the client and distribute a comprehensive list of medications with detailed information regarding dosages, functions, and implications (**Table 2**).

Treatment

As volume status is of the utmost concern, the client will be on diuretics for fluid volume preload management. Loop and thiazide diuretics are often used but can precipitate hypokalemia. As such, potassium is supplemented to prevent corresponding arrhythmias from deficiencies. Less frequently a potassium-sparing diuretic, such as spironolactone may be used.[9,16,17]

To decrease the workload of the heart, the cardiologist often orders afterload reduction agents. ACE inhibitors such as enalapril, captopril, or lisinopril selectively suppress the renin–angiotensin–aldosterone system, inhibit ACE, and prevent the angiotensin I to angiotensin II conversion. Because they are effective antihypertensive agents, initial doses may precipitate hypotension. If used with diuretics they may cause hyperkalemia or elevation in kidney dysfunction.[9,18]

By selectively blocking the vasoconstrictor and aldosterone-secreting effects of angiotensin II, angiotensin receptor blockers, such as losartan or valsartan, are an alternative for those with hypersensitivity that cannot tolerate the abovementioned ACE inhibitors. In rare cases, both may lead to angioedema, renal failure, or thrombocytopenia.[9,17,18]

In the absence of a respiratory disease contraindication, beta-blockers such as metoprolol or carvedilol reduce afterload by decreasing heart rate and increasing stroke volumes. They reduce elevated renin plasma levels and block beta-2 adrenergic smooth muscle receptors.

By blocking depolarization calcium influx, coronary and vascular smooth muscles dilate by calcium channel blockers such as felodipine, nifedipine, or amlodipine.

Table 2
Medications

	Indication	Implications	Contraindication	Side Effects
Furosemide	Preload management	Edema	Anuria Hypovolemia	Hypokalemia
Hydrochlorothiazide	Preload management	Edema	Anuria Thiazide sensitivity	Renal dysfunction
Spironolactone	Diuretic	Potassium sparing	Hyperkalemia	Secondary malignancy
Enalapril	Afterload reduction	Suppresses the renin-angiotensin-aldosterone system	History of angioedema	Hypotension Renal dysfunction Neutropenia Angioedema
Captopril	Antihypertensive	ACE inhibitor	Hypersensitivity	Angioedema Renal failure Death
Losartan	Antihypertensive	Blocks angiotensin II vasoconstriction	Hypersensitivity	Angioedema Renal failure Thrombocytopenia
Valsartan	Antihypertensive	Blocks angiotensin II vasoconstriction	Hepatic disease Renal artery stenosis	Second-degree AV block
Lisinopril	Antihypertensive	ACE inhibitor	Hypersensitivity	Angioedema
Metoprolol	Reduce afterload	Block beta-2 adrenergic smooth muscle receptors Reduce elevated renin plasma levels	COPD	Respiratory exacerbation
Carvedilol	Antihypertensive	Nonselective alpha/beta blocker	COPD Second- or third-degree heart block	AV block Pulmonary edema
Felodipine	Calcium channel blocker	Block depolarization calcium influx dilating vascular smooth muscles	Second- and third-degree heart blocks Pulmonary congestion Acute MI	Dysrhythmias
Nifedipine	Calcium channel blocker	Block depolarization calcium influx dilating vascular smooth muscles	Cardiogenic shock	Dysrhythmias
Amlodipine	Calcium channel blocker	Block depolarization calcium influx dilating vascular smooth muscles	Severe aortic stenosis	Flushing Peripheral edema

Abbreviations: AV, atrioventricular; COPD, chronic obstructive pulmonary disease; MI, myocardial infarction.

They are contraindicated in second- and third-degree heart blocks, pulmonary congestion, or acute myocardial infarction.[9,18]

Arteriole smooth muscles are directly relaxed by vasodilators such as hydralazine or labetalol. Blood pressures are reduced with subsequent increases in stroke volume, cardiac output, and heart rate.[5,9]

By inhibiting sodium-potassium ATPase, digoxin potentiates calcium for cardiac contractility. Cardiac output increases as the contraction force increases with the positive inotropic effect. Likewise atria-ventricular conduction and heart rates decrease.[9,17,18]

For hemodynamically unstable patients dobutamine agonizes beta-1 receptors while increasing cardiac output. Response dosage titration is used to increase contractility while monitoring for excessive tachycardia riposte from the cardiac stimulant effect. Causing mesenteric and renal dilation at low-dose intravenous dopamine decreases afterload as well as increases cardiac output with beta-1 inotropic stimulation.[7]

Because the associated arrhythmia is usually atrial fibrillation, digoxin is often ordered for heart rate control. Considering the increased likelihood of clot formation from dysfunctional cardiac blood flow associated with valvular heart disease, clients are prescribed anticoagulants. They will need information concerning bleeding risks, nutritional implications, monitoring, and interactions.[3,6]

Education

As medication, compliance is ultimately important for maintenance and survival and nurses must thoroughly educate their clients on risk, administration recommendations as well as dietary implications. Anticoagulants may require specific sequential testing and adjustment titrations. Those taking digoxin will need to learn to take their pulse as well as a staggering administration schedule if they are taking antacids. Because many antihypertensive and diuretic medications may be nephrotoxic, they will need interval metabolic laboratory studies for surveillance. Likewise, clients will need to be well versed on signs of toxicity or overmedication such as confusion, dizziness, or weakness.

Before dental or respiratory invasive procedures clients are recommended to take prophylactic antibiotic to prevent bacterial infiltration and colonization on the compromised valvular intima surfaces. Likewise, any open wounds require prompt attention that includes cleansing and appropriate antibiotic topical agents.[13,19]

Clients will need to be well versed on the manifestations of worsening heart disease. They should know to promptly report weight gains of 3 pounds in 1 day or 5 pounds in 1 week. Signs of worsening dyspnea, fatigue, nausea, vomiting, cough, edema, syncope, decreased urine output, or changes in their blood pressure maintenance should be shared with the support staff for urgent evaluation of possible hospitalization for stabilization and treatment.[4,9,11]

Interdisciplinary Approach

Because lifestyle modification related to cholesterol and weight management are essential, dietary services may be consulted to provide counsel and individual recommendations. Respiratory services may be needed to facilitate nebulizer management, supplemental oxygen therapy if indicated, and incentive spirometry education. Clients with prolonged weakness may require rehabilitative services to facilitate restoration of activity levels.

Nursing Implications

The nurse is involved in every aspect of the comprehensive care of the valvular patient. In addition to the direct care involved in hospitalization and surgical episodes, the nurse empowers the client directing self-management and collaborates the contributing disciplines. The education components include medications, disease characteristics, compliance, and dietary recommendations. The nurse encourages independence and increasing levels of activity to increase cardiovascular fitness. The client is educated about progressive tolerance as well as manifestation on which to report immediately.

Few studies have begun to quantify client behavior modification in response to such structure. Ramya and Andrews cite increased effectiveness with family involvement and structured protocol teaching manifested in higher compliance, more exercise, and fewer problems after their cardiac valve surgery.[20] Many research opportunities immerge as nurses look at how to most effectively affect client care and outcomes.

SUMMARY

As the population ages, the development of valvular heart disease becomes more likely. With aggressive medical management to control hypertension and dyslipidemia, onset of escalating valve malfunction and corresponding symptomology may be delayed. In addition to innovative surgical repair and replacement, vastly improving cardiac function, there is still much to learn about the effective titration balance to improve client outcomes, mortality, and quality of life.

REFERENCES

1. Linden B. The management of valvular heart disease. Brit J of Card Nur 2013; 8(2):60–2.
2. Erdi J, Sydo N, Sydo T, et al. Prognostic significance of heart rate recovery valvular heart disease. J Am Coll Cardiol 2018;71:A2021–9.
3. Abraham W, Vahanian A, Alfiere O, et al. Transcatheter mitral valve repair in patients with functional mitral regurgitation – one-year outcomes from the multicenter CE trial. J Card Fail 2017;23(11):830.
4. Nishimura RA, Otto CM, Bonow RO, et al. 2014 AHA/ACC guideline for the management of patients with valvular heart disease. J Am Coll Cardiol 2014;63(22): 57–185.
5. Kanwar A, Thaden J, Nkomo VT. Management of patients with aortic valve stenosis. Mayo Clin Proc 2018;93(4):488–508.
6. Rieck AE, Cramariuc D, Boman K. Hypertension in aortic stenosis: implications for left ventricular structure and cardiovascular events. Hypertension 2012;60: 90–7.
7. Meyer S, Suri R, Wright S, et al. Does metabolic syndrome influence bioprosthetic mitral valve degeneration and reoperation rate. J Card Surg 2012;27:146–51.
8. Ito S, Miranda W, Nkomo VT, et al. Reduced left ventricular ejection fraction in patients with aortic stenosis. J Am Coll Cardiol 2018;71(12):1313–21.
9. Bouleti C, Iung B, Himbert D, et al. Long-term efficacy of percutaneous mitral commissurotomy for restenosis after previous mitral commissurotomy. Heart 2013;99(18):1336–41.
10. Zhang H, Zhu K, Yang S, et al. Bicuspid aortic valve with critical coarctation of the aorta. J Thorac Dis 2018;10(7):4353–9.

11. Mordi I, Tzemos N. Bicuspid aortic valve disease: a comprehensive review. Cardiol Res Pract 2012;2012:196037.
12. Eleid MF, Nishimura RA, Ryan J, et al. Left ventricular diastolic dysfunction in patients with mitral stenosis undergoing percutaneous mitral balloon valvotomy. Mayo Clin Proc 2013;88(4):337–44.
13. Mutlak D, Carasso S, Lessick J, et al. Excessive respiratory variation in tricuspid regurgitation systolic velocities in patients with severe tricuspid regurgitation. Eur Heart J Cardiovasc Imaging 2013;14(10):957–62.
14. Nascimento BR, Athayde GR, Junqueira L, et al. Increased left atrial compliance is an independent predictor of improved functional capacity after percutaneous mitral valvuloplasty. J Am Coll Cardiol 2017;69:1136.
15. Thomas KL, Jackson LR, Shrader P, et al. Prevalence, characteristics, and outcomes of valvular heart disease in patients with atrial fibrillation: insights from the outcomes registry for vetter informed treatment for atrial fibrillation. J Am Heart Assoc 2017;6:1–12.
16. Nauta JF, Hummel YM, van der Meer P, et al. Correlation with invasive left ventricular filling pressures and prognostic relevance of the echocardiographic diastolic parameters used in the 2016 ESC heart failure guidelines and in the 2016 ASE/EACVI recommendations. Eur J Heart Fail 2018;20(9):1303–11.
17. Vassileva CM, Mishkel G, McNeely C. Long-term survival of patients undergoing mitral valve repair and replacement: a longitudinal analysis of Medicare fee-for-service beneficiaries. Circulation 2013;127:1870–6.
18. Vahanian A, Alfiere O, Andreotti F. Guidelines on the management of valvular heart disease (version 2012). Eur Heart J 2012;33:2451–96.
19. Michelena HI, Khanna AD, Mahoney D, et al. Incidence of aortic complications in patients with bicuspid aortic valves. JAMA 2011;306(10):1104–12.
20. Ramya KR, Andrews GR. Efffectiveness of discharge counseling on compliance and problems of patients who have undergone heart valve replacement. International J Nur Edu 2012;4(1):49–51.

Cardiovascular Disease Management in Minority Women: Special Considerations

Latanja Lawrence Divens, PhD, DNP, APRN, FNP-BC[a],*,
Benita N. Chatmon, PhD, MSN, RN[b]

KEYWORDS

- Racial/ethnic minorities • Hypertension • Diabetes • Health care disparities
- Overweight/obesity

KEY POINTS

- Black women have a higher prevalence of cardiovascular disease than any other ethnic minority group.
- To prevent cardiovascular disease, women should eat a heart-healthy diet, maintain an active lifestyle, maintain normal blood pressure and cholesterol levels, and refrain from tobacco use.
- A multilayered approach of prevention and management strategies impacting physical, mental, and social well-being is needed to improve the health of minority women.

INTRODUCTION

Cardiovascular disease (CVD) is one of the leading killers of Americans. In fact, CVD has become one of the costliest chronic diseases in the nation. In the past, CVD usually resulted in death. However, with the increase in research and modification of life style behaviors (eg, abstinence from smoking, adoption of a healthy diet, and increase in exercise), as well as improved emergency response, a decline in CVD occurred between the years 2001 and 2011. However, in the past few years, progress came to a halt.[1]

CVD used to be known to occur primarily in men.[2] Along with the higher prevalence, men also died from CVD in the mid-20th century. With the increase of incidence of CVD in women, data from men's mortality rates are being used as a preventive measure for the CVD occurring in women.[3] The mortality rate is being increasingly recognized as a preventable epidemic that occurs in women. CVD in women is among

Disclosure Statement: The authors have nothing to declare.
[a] School of Nursing, LSU Health New Orleans, 1900 Gravier Street, Office, New Orleans, LA 70112, USA; [b] School of Nursing, LSU Health New Orleans, 1900 Gravier Street, Office 331, New Orleans, LA 70112, USA
* Corresponding author.
E-mail address: ldive1@lsuhsc.edu

Crit Care Nurs Clin N Am 31 (2019) 39–47
https://doi.org/10.1016/j.cnc.2018.11.004
0899-5885/19/© 2018 Elsevier Inc. All rights reserved.

the deadliest diseases in the United States, with a mortality rate 10 times greater than that of breast cancer.[4–6] Acute myocardial infarction (MI), stroke, heart failure, hypertensive disease, and vascular disease all fall under cardiovascular diseases. Each year, approximately 225,000 women over the age of 84 will die from heart disease compared with 50,000 deaths from cancer.[7]

Similarly, the Centers for Disease Control and Prevention (CDC) reported that during a 27-year period (1979-2006), cardiac-related deaths decreased in men significantly, while there was only a moderate decline in women. In 2006 and 2007, a total of approximately 622,000 women died of heart disease alone, even with the slight decline between years.[6] One possible reason for the moderate decline of CVD in women may be because of the failure of identifying at-risk women.[7] Even with this alarming statistic, only 54% of women recognized that they were at a significant risk for cardiovascular disease. Most of the 46% of women who did not recognize the significant risk of CVD belonged to a minority group.[3,4] In fact, Morris and colleagues[8] (2018) conducted original research on race and sex differences in association to atherosclerotic CVD (ASCVD) risk and healthy lifestyle behaviors. The findings of the study concluded that minorities are less likely to engage in healthier lifestyle modifications despite higher body mass index (BMI) and ASCVD risk.

Although CVD is highly modifiable, it continues to affect racial/ethnic subgroups such as blacks, Hispanics, American Indians, Alaskan Natives, Asian Indians, and Filipinos. Minorities make up 36% of the general population and are predicted to increase to 53% by the year 2050.[9] Yet, approximately 48% of black women are burdened with increased cases of CVD related deaths than their white counterparts.[9–11] Similarly, Hispanics, American Indians, and Alaska Natives have a high prevalence of CVD. This disparity may be because of various socioeconomic and health care barriers among these minority groups.[7]

The purpose of this article is to raise awareness among minority women, particular black women, on the prevalence of CVD. An additional goal is to provide a review of the implications of identifying the major risk factors that affect this vulnerable population and the management of those risk factors.

RISK FACTORS OF CARDIOVASCULAR DISEASE

Large benefits are seen when multiple CVD risk factors are addressed.[10] Women have a higher prevalence of CVD risk factors than men except for the risk factor of smoking.[5] Risk factors are either modifiable or nonmodifiable. Modifiable risk factors are factors that can be altered or prevented, while non-modifiable risk factors are factors that cannot be prevented and are usually something innate.[6] Some examples of modifiable risk factors for CVD are diabetes mellitus, history of smoking, lack of physical activity, overweight/obesity, hypertension, hyperlipidemia, and a stroke. Modifiable risk factors can be controlled by taking up a healthier lifestyle that involves diet and exercise, as well as medication management. Nonmodifiable risk factors include age, genetics, gender, and ethnicity. Although one cannot change his or her genetics or gender, he or she can make provisions to reduce chances of developing CVD by initiating healthy lifestyle changes.

Various aspects of cardiovascular health in minority women have been studied, and research has identified that obesity and hypertension rates are highest among black women when compared with all other racial/ethnic groups combined.[12] Four out of 5 black women are considered obese. One in 4 black women over the age of 55 have diabetes mellitus.[11] Understanding how to prevent or reduce CVD risk factors could drastically decrease the mortality rate among minorities with CVD.

THE IMPACT OF ATHEROSCLEROSIS AND INFLAMMATION ON HYPERTENSION, DIABETES, HYPERLIPIDEMIA, AND OBESITY

The risk of cardiovascular disease for minority women is greatest among black women with inflammatory, dietary, and behavior-related diseases, with conditions including hypertension, stroke, and obesity being some of the most common.[13] The prevalence of these conditions significantly increases the risk of CVD, as these conditions support the development of endothelial dysfunction, often leading to the development of atherosclerosis. Atherosclerosis is a multifactorial and complex disease in which inflammation plays a role in all stages of the disease process.[14] Atherosclerosis is now considered a systemic disease featuring low-grade arterial inflammatory lesions that can develop through the disease progression.[15] Endothelial cell dysfunction is impacted by stress and results in inflammatory or oxidative stress and injury, impaired glucose, hyperlipidemia (HLD), and hypertension (HTN).[14,16]

The 2007 update on guidelines for the prevention of CVD included 3 categories of risk (at high risk, at risk, and at optimal risk). These classifications were based several observations:

- Prevention is extremely important in all women despite their ethnicity, because the lifetime risk of CVD in women is boisterous.
- Almost all the clinical trials data used to create the recommendations were based on women who were high risk for CVD or relatively healthy with a minute amount of risk.
- There were limitations noted that may have affected how women were categorized based on their risk scores. Some of those limitations include the focus on a short-term risk within a 10-year period, lack of familial history, incorrect statistics on prevalence of the nonwhite population, and the notion that subclinical CVD can have a higher prevalence among women categorized as low risk.[2]

The updated 2011 guidelines have since added to the criteria of each of the risk categories (**Table 1**) based on the noted observations. In addition, ideal cardiovascular recommendations were added (**Table 2**) to the guidelines.[1,2]

Atherosclerosis

Atherosclerosis is a complex process of vascular remodeling and restructuring that includes an inflammatory process, and hardening and narrowing of arteries because of a

Table 1	
Cardiovascular disease risk factors	
Diseases and Behaviors	**Recommendations to Reduce Risk**
Diabetes	HgbA1C <7.0 mg/dl
Tobacco Use	Abstinence from tobacco use
Hypertension	Blood Pressure <120/<80 mm Hg
Poor Exercise	150 min per week of moderate-intensity aerobic activity or 75 min per week of vigorous aerobic activity
Poor Diet	Follow a low fat, low-salt diet such a Mediterranean or DASH diet (**Table 2**)
Obesity	BMI <25 kg/m^2

Data from Mosca L, Benjamin E, Berra K, et al. Effectiveness-based guidelines for the prevention of cardiovascular disease in women–2011 update: a guideline from the American Heart Association. Circulation 2011;123(11):1243–62.

Table 2
Dietary patterns to reduce cardiovascular risk

Dietary Approaches to Stop Hypertension (DASH) Pattern	Mediterranean-Style Diet (MED) Pattern
Diet high in: • Vegetables • Fruits • Low-fat dairy products • Whole grains • Poultry • Fish • Nuts Low in: • Sweets • Sugar-sweetened beverages • Red meats. The DASH dietary pattern is • High in potassium, magnesium, and calcium • High in protein and fiber.	Diet higher in: • Fruits (fresh) • Vegetables (root and green varieties) • Whole grains (cereals, breads, rice, or pasta) • Fatty fish (rich in omega–3 fatty acids) Lower in: • Red meat (emphasizing lean meats) The MED Pattern: • High in fiber (27–37 g/d) • High in polyunsaturated fatty acids

Data from Mosca L, Benjamin E, Berra K, et al. Effectiveness-based guidelines for the prevention of cardiovascular disease in women–2011 update: a guideline from the American Heart Association. Circulation 2011;123(11):1243–62.

build-up of cholesterols, fats, and other substances on the inside of arterial walls. The disease is multifactorial and complex, in which inflammation plays a role in all stages of the disease process.[14] Atherosclerosis is now considered a systemic disease, featured by low-grade arterial inflammatory lesions that can develop through the disease progression.[15] Endothelial cell dysfunction is impacted by stress and results in inflammatory or oxidative stress and injury, impaired glucose, hyperlipidemia (HLD), and HTN.[14,16] Atherosclerosis is highly prevalent in minority populations in the United States. Effects of the disease include but are not limited to acute coronary syndrome, carotid stenosis, angina, and peripheral vascular disease.[14,16]

Hypertension

HTN is the most common risk factor for CVD, especially among the minority population. The complexities of managing HTN have been a great challenge among health care providers. A higher percentage of women than men have high blood pressure after the age of 65. In addition, black women have the highest prevalence of HTN in the world. Between 1988 and 2002, the prevalence of HTN in blacks increased from 36% to 41%. More disturbingly, it was higher among black women than black men.[2]

HTN occurs when the force needed for blood flow through the blood vessels is too high.[17] When high blood pressure is left untreated, significant risk for strokes, chronic kidney disease, and other health conditions can occur. The 2017 Guideline for High Blood Pressure in Adults (2017-GHBP), developed by the American College of Cardiology and the American Heart Association, classifies blood pressure in 4 stages: normal, elevated, stage 1, and stage 2, with the goal blood pressure being a systolic blood pressure of 120 mm Hg systolic and a diastolic blood pressure of 80 mm Hg (**Table 3**).[1] The 2017-GHBP neglects the recommendations of the Eighth National Report of the Joint National Committee on Prevention, Detection, Evaluation, and Treatment of High Blood Pressure (JNC-8). The 2017-GHBP therefore is an update of JNC-7 and recommends lower blood pressures for all adult populations to reduce

Table 3 2017 high blood pressure guidelines			
Blood Pressure Category	**Systolic**	**Diastolic**	**Recommendations**
Normal	<120Hg	<80 mm Hg	No modifications required/continue to maintain healthy lifestyle
Elevated	120–129 mm Hg	>80 mm Hg	Lifestyle modifications
Hypertension			
Stage 1	130–139 mm Hg Or	80–89 mm Hg	Lifestyle modifications Pharmacologic therapy
Stage 2	≥140 mm Hg Or	≥90 mm Hg	Lifestyle modifications Pharmacologic therapy usually requiring 2 medications

Data from Whelton PK, Carey RM, Aronow WS, et al. 2017 ACC/AHA/AAPA/ABC/ACPM/AGS/APhA/ ASH/ASPC/NMA/PCNA guideline for the prevention, detection, evaluation, and management of high blood pressure in adults: a report of the American College of Cardiology/American Heart Association task force on clinical practice guidelines. J Am Coll Cardiol 2018;71:e127–248.

the risk of the development of CVD. The Multi-Ethnic Study of Atherosclerosis (MESA), 2018, a medical research study conducted by the National Heart, Lung and Blood Institute, was initiated in 1999 and continues to be ongoing. MESA examines early or subclinical atherosclerosis. Findings from MESA provide support for the 2017-GHBP guideline as black and Hispanic populations have been identified as having a higher lifetime risk of developing HTN and CVD.[13]

HTN is associated with accelerated atherosclerosis and loss of the endothelium's ability to modulate vascular relaxation mediated by nitric oxide. Vascular tone and reactivity are continuously regulated by endothelial cells that normally respond to neurohormonal and mechanical factors with physiologic and pathologic conditions.[14] The endothelium responds to physiologic and pathologic changes by releasing relaxing and contracting mediators including nitric oxide, prostacyclin, and endothelium-derived hyperpolarizing factor.[14] These mediators contribute to the loss of the modulatory role of the endothelium and result in endothelial dysfunction and hypertension that occurs because of the increased arterial pressure related to the increased peripheral resistance and the contractile state of the resistant arteries; the release of inflammatory biomarkers and endothelial dysfunction drives this process.[16]

Hyperlipidemia

Black women have been identified as a population at increased risk for CVD, with hyperlipidemia being a major risk factor. Hyperlipidemia is most often managed with a combination of nonpharmacologic and pharmacologic therapies. Yet research has identified that black women are treated less aggressively, often not being prescribed a statin, while white men received the most rigorous treatment of all groups.[18] It is estimated that 36.1% of black women and 42% of Hispanic women are diagnosed with hyperlipidemia; the elevation of blood cholesterol, triglycerides, or both is a clear risk factor for the development of atherosclerosis.[19]

Cholesterol, most commonly known for its pathogenic properties, also has an important role in the modulation of cell membrane fluidity and hormone synthesis. Low-grade chronic inflammation has been identified as a major insult to this process and encourages the development of atherosclerosis and coronary heart disease. The induction of the inflammatory process may substantiate and provide a linkage between hyperlipidemia and atherogenesis.[19] The fatty acid profile of the phospholipids mirrors the cell membrane's composition, which impacts the cell membrane's ability to regulate the inflammatory process.[15]

Adult Obesity

Adult obesity is a common condition in minority women, with an estimated 82% of black women age 20 and older being overweight or obese in comparison to 61% of white women.[13] Adult obesity is defined as a BMI of 30.0 kg/m^2 or greater.[20] The condition is associated with chronic, low-level inflammation and hormone and metabolic dysfunction.[20] Adipose tissue is no longer viewed as fat storage cells but is now known to function in metabolic control and as an endocrine organ. Adipose tissue has 4 major functions, including: serving as repositories of free fatty acids (FFAs), hormone regulation, which is impacted by weight gain and results in dysregulation of metabolic functions and inflammation, and as a regulator of FFA storage and oxidation in adipocytes and the periphery.[21] Dysregulation of adipose tissue and adiposopathy, the pathogenic enlargement of adipose cells and tissue, are linked to the local inflammatory processes where inflamed adipose tissue produces tumor necrosis factor (TNF) and other cytokines that leak into circulation and result in systemic inflammation and impaired cellular metabolism. C-reactive protein is the primary acute phase reactant of this systemic, inflammatory response.[21] The effects of adiposopathy and systemic inflammation are fueled by an elevated BMI and can lead to the development of cardiovascular and metabolic diseases[21]

Physical Activity and Exercise

Black women have been identified as the least active group when compared with other groups of women, specifically whites and Hispanics, and are found to be less likely to participate in behaviors that reduce CVD risk such as a low-fat, and low sodium diet, exercise, and a physical activity regimen.[13] This reality, coupled with data from evaluations of health interventions, demonstrates that black women are less likely to benefit from strategies currently utilized to improve CVD risks.[13] Evaluations of the effectiveness of the current strategies have forced the consideration of the impact of cultural influence, time and schedule constraints, adherence issues, and the available resources to support behavior changes in black women. Additionally, a lack of awareness about preventive health and supportive strategies, including a lack of support for black women to encourage buy in to physical activity and lifestyle modifications to support cardiovascular health exists. There are several additional areas of concern that must be considered:

- Failure of health care providers to discuss the impact of exercise and daily/weekly activity needs
- Failure of the health care communities to offer opportunities that encourage preventive health care
- Repeated missed opportunities to engage black women in interventions to encourage physical activity.[13]

The African American Collaborative Obesity Research Network (AACORN) encourages the establishment of collaborative partnerships to engage the community and stakeholders in the development and implementation phases of strategies to support weight loss. AACORN also stresses the need to consider cultural and social processes, economic status, and the physical environments of minorities in the planning and development of health-promoting activities. Consideration of these factors is essential to the process and will support adherence and engagement of participants.[13]

Diabetes

Type 2 diabetes mellitus (T2DM) is a progressive, chronic disorder characterized by insulin resistance and beta-cell dysfunction.[20] The defining feature of the condition is chronic, mild inflammation driven by proinflammatory cytokines.[14] Glucose homeostasis is regulated by hormones including but not limited to insulin, amylin, leptin, and glucagon.[14] Insulin regulates fat and protein metabolism and intracellular transport of glucose. Hyperglycemia results in oxidative stress and endothelial dysfunction.[14] Atherosclerosis is accelerated in T2DM, with prolonged exposure to hyperglycemia leading to increased nitric oxide synthase, resulting in endothelial dysfunction.[14,15]

THE IMPACT OF HEALTH CARE DISPARITIES ON CARDIOVASCULAR DISEASE IN MINORITY WOMEN

The demographics of the United States are changing. It is getting more diverse, so that health care professionals will have to consider diversity to improve the quality of care and reduce health care disparities. Factors that should be considered when combating disparities include socioeconomic status, race, lack of awareness, lack of accessible care, occupational status, religious affiliation, culture, and gender, to name a few.[2,12] CVD affects black and Hispanic women at disproportionate rates compared with white women.[7,11] Socioeconomic status also contributes to the prevalence of CVD. Often the disadvantaged populations are either uninsured or underinsured and usually belong to a minority group therefore, contributing to limited access to health care.[6]

PREVENTIVE HEALTH STRATEGIES

Prevention and strategies to improve the health of black women should be multilayered and include strategies that will impact physical, mental, and social well-being. Research has demonstrated the usefulness and impact of programs that are culturally tailored to improve cardiovascular-related health outcomes.[13] Mind-body therapies (MBTs), physical activity and health education strategies will provide a comprehensive approach for minority women.

HEALTH EDUCATION

CVD-related knowledge has improved for minority women over the last 15 years; however, many minority women still lack knowledge about cardiovascular-related risk factors, mortality, preventive measures, and complications.[16] In a study of ethnic minority women, researchers sought to identify specific culturally sensitive needs regarding health-promoting behaviors and CVD[13] Black and Hispanic women were found to be less likely to be aware of heart disease than white women in addition to health-promoting strategies to improve health and decrease risks. When considering the impact of cultural influence on the health of black women, it is important to recognize how black women prioritize health. It has been found that black women prioritize health differently from other populations. For black women, psychological health/well-being is the first health-related priority, followed by financial and physical health, respectively.[11] It is therefore imperative that these realities be considered when developing health-promotion strategies for this population to address the unique needs and priorities of this population. Incorporating MBTs is therefore essential to protect and promote the health of black women.[13]

DIETARY MODIFICATIONS

Dietary modification are also a topic that must be considered thoroughly when educating minority women. Providing education on the Dietary Approaches to Stop Hypertension (DASH) will likely not consider cultural methods of food preparation, as the use of salt and salt-containing seasonings or spices in moderation is challenging. Blacks have frequently been identified as low adopters of low-salt diets, which challenges this recommendation. The AACORN identified that the use of groups that work together to achieve common goals to support change also supports individual behavior change.[13] Incorporating strategies that support lifestyle modifications including food preparation and selection may have significant impact on behavior change when offered in a culturally sensitive manner.

PHYSICAL ACTIVITY AND MIND–BODY THERAPIES

Strategies to improve health and reduce stress include various activities such as daily scheduled exercise (eg, walking, running, jogging, or cycling) and MBTs. MBTs are adjunctive health care strategies used to support conventional care. It is estimated that 30% of the adults in the United States participate in some form of MBT. MBTs improve an individual's feelings of well-being and reduces psychological and systemic stress on the body.[12] Examples of MBT include yoga, tai chi, qi gong, deep breathing and meditation.[12] See the American College of Cardiology and American Heart Association's recommendations for physical activity for adults (see **Table 3**). When providing culturally competent care for minority women, it is important educate, encourage, involve, and support this population to make the best decisions to support health in a social context.

SUMMARY

There is a clear need to educate minority women on prevention and management of risk factors that lead to CVD. Black women have the highest prevalence of CVD. HTN, diabetes, overweight/obesity, smoking, and hyperlipidemia have shown some correlation to the prevalence of CVD among minorities. Therefore, implementing strategies to increase awareness, and to prevent and manage CVD risk factors, is vital.

REFERENCES

1. American College of Cardiology, American Heart Association. 2017 guideline for high blood pressure in adults - American College of Cardiology. Am Coll Cardiol 2017. Available at: http://www.acc.org/latest-in-cardiology/ten-points-to-remember/2017/11/09/11/41/2017-guideline-for-high-blood-pressure-in-adults. Accessed June 30, 2018.

2. Mosca L, Benjamin E, Berra K, et al. Effectiveness-based guidelines for the prevention of cardiovascular disease in women–2011 update: a guideline from the American Heart Association. Circulation 2011;123(11):1243–62.

3. Limacher M, Bavry A. Prevention of cardiovascular disease in women. Semin Reprod Med 2014;32(06):447–53.

4. National Center for Chronic Disease Prevention and Health Promotion. Division for heart disease and stroke prevention. Women and heart disease fact Sheet|Data & Statistics|DHDSP|CDC. CDCgov.. 2017. Available at: https://www.cdc.gov/dhdsp/data_statistics/fact_sheets/fs_women_heart.htm. Accessed June 27, 2018.

5. Farmer G, Jabson J, Bucholz K, et al. A population-based study of cardiovascular disease risk in sexual-minority women. Am J Public Health 2013;103(10): 1845–50.
6. Vaid I, Wigington C, Borbely D, et al. WISEWOMAN: addressing the needs of women at high risk for cardiovascular disease. J Womens Health 2011;20(7): 977–82.
7. Bullock-Palmer R. Prevention, detection and management of coronary artery disease in minority females. Ethn Dis 2015;25(4):499.
8. Morris A, Ko Y, Hutcheson S, et al. Race/ethnic and sex differences in the association of atherosclerotic cardiovascular disease risk and healthy lifestyle behaviors. J Am Heart Assoc 2018;7(10):e008250.
9. Frank A, Zhao B, Jose P, et al. Racial/ethnic differences in dyslipidemia patterns. Circulation 2013;129(5):570–9.
10. American Diabetes Association. Cardiovascular disease and risk management. Diabetes Care 2014;38(Supplement_1):S49–57.
11. Belgrave F, Abrams J. Reducing disparities and achieving equity in African American women's health. Am Psychol 2016;71(8):723–33.
12. Johnson C, Sheffield K, Brown R. Mind-body therapies for African-American women at risk for cardiometabolic disease: a systematic review. Evid Based Complement Alternat Med 2018;2018:1–11.
13. Brown A, Hudson L, Chui K, et al. Improving heart health among black/African American women using civic engagement: a pilot study. BMC Public Health 2017;17(1). https://doi.org/10.1186/s12889-016-3964-2.
14. Cosentino F, Lüscher T. Effects of blood pressure and glucose on endothelial function. Curr Hypertens Rep 2001;3(1):79–88.
15. Dessì M, Noce A, Bertucci P, et al. Atherosclerosis, dyslipidemia, and inflammation: the significant role of polyunsaturated fatty acids. ISRN Inflamm 2013;2013: 1–13.
16. Villablanca A, Warford C, Wheeler K. Inflammation and cardiometabolic risk in African American women is reduced by a pilot community-based educational intervention. J Womens Health 2016;25(2):188–99.
17. American Heart Association. The facts about high blood pressure. Heartorg 2018. Available at: http://www.heart.org/HEARTORG/Conditions/HighBlood Pressure/GettheFactsAboutHighBloodPressure/The-Facts-About-High-Blood-Pressure_UCM_002050_Article.jsp. Accessed June 27, 2018.
18. Safford M, Gamboa C, Durant R, et al. Race–sex differences in the management of hyperlipidemia. Am J Prev Med 2015;48(5):520–7.
19. Gulati M, Noel Bairey Merz C. New cholesterol guidelines and primary prevention in women. Trends Cardiovasc Med 2015;25(2):84–94.
20. Denis G, Sebastiani P, Bertrand K, et al. Inflammatory signatures distinguish metabolic health in African-American women with obesity. PLoS One 2018; 13(5):e0196755.
21. American Heart Association. Obesity and cardiovascular disease risk. Cardiology 2018. Available at: https://www.acc.org/latest-in-cardiology/articles/2018/07/06/12/42/cover-story-obesity-and-cardiovascular-disease-risk. Accessed October 31, 2018.

ST-Elevation Myocardial Infarction and Non-ST-Elevation Myocardial Infarction

Medical and Surgical Interventions

Deedra H. Harrington, DNP, MSN, APRN, ACNP-BC*,
Frances Stueben, DNP, MSN, RN, CCRN, CHSE,
Christy McDonald Lenahan, DNP, APRN, FNP-BC, ENP-C, CNE

KEYWORDS

- STEMI • NSTEMI • Coronary artery disease (CAD)

KEY POINTS

- Early recognition and identification of patients with STEMI or NSTEMI is vital for improved patient outcomes.
- Early treatment is indicated with adequate pharmacologic and interventional coronary reperfusion.
- Identification of appropriate treatment is the goal for limiting myocardial tissue damage.

INTRODUCTION

Coronary artery disease (CAD) is the leading cause of death in both men and women among most ethnic and racial groups in the United States.[1] Every 40 seconds one American suffers from a myocardial infarction (MI). Annually, Americans experience 790,000 MIs, 580,000 being first time MIs and 210,000 subsequent MIs.[2] Over time, however, with early recognition and treatment the incidence of MI has demonstrated a significant decline.[3]

RISK FACTORS FOR CORONARY ARTERY DISEASE

Risk factors for CAD can be categorized into nonmodifiable and modifiable. Nonmodifiable risk factors include age of more than 45 years in men and more than 55 years in women; family history of early heart disease; and African American race.[4] Modifiable risk factors include hypercholesterolemia, specifically related to elevation of

Disclosure Statement: The authors have nothing to disclose.
Department of Nursing, University of Louisiana at Lafayette, College of Nursing and Allied Health Professions, 411 East Street Mary Boulevard, Lafayette, LA 70504, USA
* Corresponding author.
E-mail address: deedraharrington@louisiana.edu

low-density lipoprotein cholesterols (LDL-C); hypertension; tobacco abuse; diabetes mellitus; obesity; lack of physical activity; metabolic syndrome; and/or mental distress and depression.[4] Several medical conditions are also considered risk factors for CAD (**Box 1**).[4]

PATHOPHYSIOLOGY

CAD results from endothelial dysfunction that causes a proinflammatory, prothrombotic state.[5] The ensuing atherosclerosis then leads to arterial thrombosis and possible arterial obstruction.[5] The obstructing thrombus, if formed in the coronary artery, can lead to MI.[5]

MI is diagnosed as either a ST-segment elevation (STEMI) or a non-STEMI (NSTEMI).[5] There are several events that may lead to MI (**Box 2**), but the most common pathogenesis is plaque rupture and resulting coronary artery thrombosis.[5] In NSTEMI, coronary artery thrombosis typically causes partial occlusion of the coronary artery resulting in subendocardial ischemia and necrosis.[5]

Similar to NSTEMI, STEMI is ultimately a result of plaque rupture leading to coronary artery thrombosis.[5] Unlike NSTEMI, however, the coronary artery thrombosis results in total occlusion of the coronary artery and extensive ischemia and necrosis that extends from the endocardium to the epicardium (ie, transmural ischemia).[5]

SIGNS AND SYMPTOMS

Signs and symptoms of NSTEMI and STEMI are similar and diagnosis is not differentiated until an electrocardiogram (ECG) has been completed. Chest pain is typically described as a heaviness or pressure lasting more than 20 minutes and present at rest.[6] Patients often complain of pain radiating to the left arm, left shoulder, neck, or jaw.[6] Diaphoresis, nausea, vomiting, dyspnea, palpitations, syncope, or near syncope may also be present in patients experiencing NSTEMI/STEMI.[6] Women, the elderly, and patients with chronic disease such as diabetes mellitus may have atypical presentations and often complain of dyspnea and/or indigestion rather than actual chest pain when experiencing NSTEMI/STEMI.[6]

DIAGNOSIS
Electrocardiogram

Considering the need for urgent intervention in the presence of STEMI, the ECG is the most important tool in initial evaluation of patients suspected of having acute MI.[7]

Box 1
Medical condition risk factors for coronary artery disease

- End-stage renal disease
- Lupus
- Rheumatoid arthritis
- Human immunodeficiency virus or AIDS
- Low serum testosterone levels
- Hysterectomy
- Xanthelasma (raised yellow patches around eyelids)

Box 2
Causes of myocardial infarction

- Plaque rupture and thrombus embolization
- Dynamic obstruction (ie, vasospasm)
- Narrowing of epicardial arteries (ie, evolving atherosclerosis, post-stent restenosis)
- Inflammatory mechanisms (ie, vasculitis)
- Extrinsic factors leading to poor coronary perfusion (hypotension, hypovolemia, or hypoxia)

Based on current guidelines published by the American College of Cardiology/American Heart Association (ACC/AHA), ECG should be obtained and interpreted by an experienced physician within 10 minutes of presentation of any patient suspected of having an MI.[8] In addition, in any patient, 45 years of age or older, with any type of chest or abdominal discomfort, ECG should be performed as part of the initial work-up.[7]

Electrocardiogram in non-ST-elevation myocardial infarction

NSTEMI, as well as unstable angina, typically cause ST-segment depressions and inverted T waves (**Fig. 1**).[9] Current guidelines indicate that diagnosis of ischemia is made when ST-segment depression is new and there is horizontal or downsloping in at least 2 anatomically contiguous leads measuring greater than or equal to 0.5 mm.[10] Criteria for ischemic T-wave inversions require inversion that is greater than or equal to 1 mm in at least 2 anatomically contiguous leads with presence of

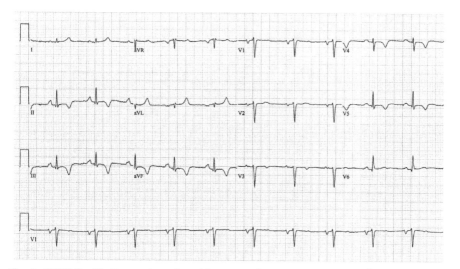

Fig. 1. NSTEMI with T-wave inversion. (*Courtesy of* Apex Innovations, Lafayette, LA; with permission.)

R waves.[10] In a small minority of patients presenting with NSTEMI, initial ECG may be normal; thus, it is important to evaluate additional factors such as history, physical examination, cardiac biomarkers, and serial ECGs before excluding a diagnosis of NSTEMI.[9]

Electrocardiogram in ST-elevation myocardial infarction

STEMI, as discussed previously, stands for ST-segment elevation MI. As its name implies, patients with STEMI will present with new ST-segment elevation in 2 anatomically contiguous leads (**Fig. 2**).[10] ST-segment elevation of greater than or equal to 1 mm in all leads except V2 and V3 is considered significant.[10] Significance of elevation in leads V2 and V3 depends on patient gender and age (**Table 1**).[10] In STEMI, presence of ST-segment elevations in specific leads illustrate where actual ischemia is occurring (**Fig. 3**).[9] Accordingly, ST-segment elevation in leads I, aVL, and V_5 to V_6 represent ischemia in the lateral wall; ST-segment elevation in leads V_2 to V_4 represent ischemia in the anterior wall; ST-segment elevation in leads II, III, and aVF represent ischemia in the inferior wall; and ST-segment elevation in leads V1 plus any other anterior leads represent ischemia in the interventricular septum.[9]

LABS

The ACC/AHA guidelines recommend troponin as the only cardiac biomarker that should be measured in patients with suspected MI.[8] Troponin, which is not normally found in serum, is only released when myocardial necrosis occurs.[8] Serial measurement 3 to 6 hours after the initial level is obtained is recommended.[7] If the initial troponin levels are negative and MI is still suspected, measurement beyond the 6-hour mark should be obtained.[7]

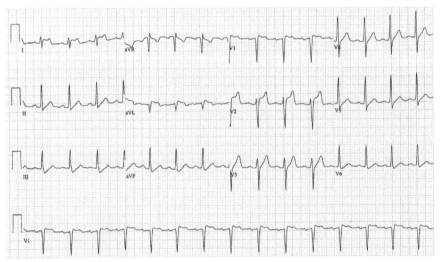

Vent. rate	93	BPM
PR interval	182	ms
QRS duration	100	ms
QT/QTc	330/410	ms
P–R–T axes	66 87	50

Fig. 2. STEMI with ST-segment elevation. (*Courtesy of* Apex Innovations, Lafayette, LA; with permission.)

Table 1
ST-segment elevation significance in leads V2 and V3

	<40 y	40 y or Older
Male	≥2.5 mm	≥2 mm
Female	≥1.5 mm	≥1.5 mm

Other laboratory studies should include a complete blood cell count, comprehensive metabolic profile, and fasting lipid profile.[7] Because of the proinflammatory state, patients with MI may have a modestly elevated white blood cell count.[7] Moreover, if the patient is going to receive a thrombolytic agent, it is important to evaluate presence of anemia as well as the platelet count.[7] Potassium and magnesium must be monitored closely in patients with MI because abnormalities can result in fatal cardiac dysrhythmias.[7] Creatinine levels are also important before specific interventions (ie, cardiac catheterization or angiotensin-converting enzyme inhibitor administration).[7]

STANDARD MEDICAL THERAPY NON-ST-ELEVATION MYOCARDIAL INFARCTION AND ST-ELEVATION MYOCARDIAL INFARCTION

Standard medical therapy and recommendations for early hospital care of NSTEMI and STEMI focus around early recognition of symptoms, reduction in ischemic injury and myocardial oxygen demand, and guided use of antiplatelet agents with timing of invasive coronary angiography.

Oxygen Therapy

Historically, oxygen therapy has been one of the initial management strategies for patients presenting with acute coronary syndrome (ACS) symptoms. Current guidelines recommend use of oxygen therapy only for patients with cyanosis, breathlessness, hypoxia (oxygen saturation <90%), or patients with heart failure (**Box 3**).[8,11] Recent data indicate that oxygen therapy in nonhypoxic patients may increase coronary vascular resistance, reduce coronary blood flow, and increase risk of mortality.[11]

Nitrates

Administration of nitrates is considered first-line medication therapy for patients who present with ACS symptoms (**Table 2**). Nitrates are helpful in the vasodilation of peripheral and coronary arteries. In addition to its vasodilation effects, nitrates also aid in the reduction of cardiac preload and reduce ventricular wall tension.[8] AHA/ACC recommends intravenous nitroglycerin in patients with heart failure, hypertension, and symptoms not relieved by sublingual nitroglycerin. Topical nitroglycerin is acceptable

I Lateral	aVR	V1 Septal	V4 Anterior
II Inferior	aVL Lateral	V2 Septal	V5 Lateral
III Inferior	aVF Inferior	V3 Anterior	V6 Lateral

Fig. 3. ECG led anatomy.

Box 3
Use of oxygen therapy

- Signs of cyanosis
- Arterial oxygen saturation less than 90%
- Respiratory distress or risk features of hypoxemia (COPD, heart failure, etc.)

Abbreviation: COPD, chronic obstructive pulmonary disease.

to intravenous nitroglycerin in patients who do not have refractory or recurrent ischemic chest pain.[8]

Caution should be used when administering nitrates to patients with hypotension, right ventricular infarction, marked bradycardia, and tachycardia and patients who have received phosphodiesterase inhibitors.[8,12] In the setting of STEMI, intravenous nitrates may be useful in treating patients during the acute phase with hypertension and heart failure.[12]

Analgesic Therapy

Intravenous morphine may be initiated for continued ischemic chest pain despite maximally administered and tolerated antiischemic agents such as nitrates.[8] The role of nonsteroidal antiinflammatory drugs has proved to be nonbeneficial in the relief of ischemic pain and may increase the risk of major adverse cardiac events (MACE).[8]

Beta-Adrenergic Blockers

Oral beta-blocker therapy (**Table 3**) should be initiated within the first 24 hours in patients who do not have any of the following: (1) signs of heart failure, (2) evidence of low-output state (systolic blood pressure of less than 90 mmHG, urine output of less than 0.5 mL/kg/h), (3) increased risk for cardiogenic shock, or (4) other contraindications to beta-blockade (eg, PR interval >0.24 seconds, second- or third-degree heart block without a cardiac pacemaker, active asthma, or reactive airway disease).[8] Contraindications to beta-blocker therapy include advanced atrioventricular block,

Table 2
Antianginal/vasodilators

Sublingual NTG	NTG every 5 min x 3 doses for continued ischemic chest pain	0.3 mg–0.4 mg every 5 min up to 3 doses
Topical NTG	Typically initially placed in hospital setting. May be substituted for intravenous NTG	0.5–2 in of ointment every 4–6 h, rotate sites Common side effects: hypotension and headache
Intravenous NTG	Unrelieved chest pain after sublingual NTG x 3	Start at 5mcg/min and titrate every 3–5 min until desired response (up to 200 mcg/min)
Contraindications	Use of nitrates with recent use of phosphodiesterase inhibitor (24–28 h)	24 h after sildenafil, vardenafil 48 h after tadalafil

Abbreviation: NTG, nitroglycerin.
Data from Skidmore-Roth L. Mosby's drug guide for nursing students. 13th edition. St Louis (MO): Elsevier; 2019.

Table 3 Beta-adrenergic blockers		
Metoprolol tartrate—short acting	5 mg IV every 2 min x 3 doses, then after 15 min, give 25–50 mg oral every 6 h × 48 h then increase to target dose.	Give with food. Taper dose over 1–2 wk to discontinue *Short acting is preferred early to allow for more rapid adjustment of dose based on patients' blood pressure and heart rate
Metoprolol succinate—long acting	100–400 mg daily for angina control	Convert over to long acting before discharge. Tablets may be cut in half but do not crush or chew. Taper dose over 1–2 wk to discontinue
Atenolol	25–50 mg twice daily	Changed from short acting to long acting once patient is tolerating short acting
Carvedilol	Start at 6.25 mg twice daily and increase every 3–10 d to 12.5 mg twice daily then to 25 mg twice daily	Titration slower monitor fluid retention, hypotension or bradycardia, give with food, taper dose over 1–2 wk to discontinue
Bisoprolol	5–20 mg daily	Taper dose over 1 wk

Abbreviation: IV, intravenous.
  * Initial introduction of metoprolol recommendations state to start with short acting metoprolol tartrate.
  Data from Skidmore-Roth L. Mosby's drug guide for nursing students. 13th edition. St Louis (MO): Elsevier; 2019.

active bronchospasm, cardiogenic shock, hypotension, and acute congestive heart failure.[8]

Antiplatelet Therapy

Aspirin (ASA) therapy is initially considered the first-line antiplatelet treatment for a patient with presentation of ACS symptoms. ASA irreversibly acetylates COX-1, which blocks the production of prostaglandins and thromboxanes. The initial dosing of 162 to 325 mg (nonenteric coated) are given on presentation.[8,12] If the individual is unable to take oral preparation then a rectal suppository dose of 600 mg is considered for administration.[13] After the initial dose of 325 mg, it is recommended to start 81 mg daily.[8]

Typically, ASA and one of the $P2Y_{12}$ inhibitors is recommended for dual antiplatelet therapy (DAPT) in patients with coronary artery disease postpercutaneous coronary intervention (PCI). $P2Y_{12}$ inhibitors should be started on admission and before PCI. Each $P2Y_{12}$ inhibitor has a loading dose followed by a maintenance dose. The maintenance dose must be adhered to for a minimum of 1 year (**Table 4**).[8,14]

Calcium Channel Blockers

Calcium channel blockers (CCBs) are used as adjunctive therapy in patients with ongoing angina despite optimal treatment with beta-blockers (**Table 5**).[8] In addition to adjunct therapy, CCBs are limited and used when patients have contraindications to beta-blockers. CCBs are not recommended in the setting of left ventricular dysfunction, increased risk of cardiogenic shock, PR interval greater than 0.24 seconds, second- or third-degree atrioventricular blocks without cardiac pacemaker support.[8]

Table 4
Recommendations for P2Y$_{12}$ therapy in patients with angiotensin-converting enzyme treated with PCI

	Clopidogrel	Prasugrel	Ticagrelor
Indications	ACS, PCI	PCI	ACS, PCI
Loading dose	600 mg	60 mg	180 mg
Maintenance	75 mg daily	10 mg daily	90 mg twice daily
	Rash	*Increase risk of bleeding in prior Stroke/TIA <60 kg ≥75 y*	*Dyspnea Bradycardia Slight increase Cr*

Abbreviations: ACS, acute coronary syndrome; Cr, creatinine; PCI, percutaneous coronary intervention; TIA, transient ischemic attack.

Data from O'Gara PT, Kushner FG, Ascheim DD, et al. 2013 ACCF/AHA guideline for the management of ST-elevation myocardial infarction. Circulation 2013;127:e362–425; and Skidmore-Roth L. Mosby's drug guide for nursing students. 13th edition. St Louis (MO): Elsevier; 2019.

Cholesterol Management

Cholesterol reduction is the key to risk reduction/stratification of heart disease and progression of coronary artery disease. Four selected patient groups would benefit from statin therapy, which include the following[15]:

- Patients with any form of clinical atherosclerotic cardiovascular disease (ASCVD)
- Patients with primary LDL-C levels of 190 mg/dL or greater
- Patient with diabetes mellitus, 40 to 75 years of age, with LDL-C levels of 70 to 189 mg/dL without clinical ASCVD
- Patients without diabetes, 40 to 75 years of age, with an estimated 10-year ASCVD risk of greater than or equal to 7.5%

Lifestyle modifications and high-intensity statin therapy are recommended on all patients with NSTEMI/STEMI, unless contraindicated, and therapy should be maintained long-term.[7] Atorvastatin 80 mg daily is considered one of a high intensity statin dosing. Caution must be taken with drugs that are metabolize via CYP3A4.[12] It is also recommended that a fasting lipid profile be collected within 24 hours of admission.[8,15]

NON-ST-ELEVATION MYOCARDIAL INFARCTION

Recommendations for treatment of patients presenting with NSTEMI include an ischemia-guided therapy (medical management) versus an early invasive coronary intervention.[8] Fibrinolytic therapy is not recommended and is potentially harmful for patients with NSTEMI. Immediate invasive coronary intervention is indicated for

Table 5
Nondihydropyridine calcium channel blockers

Diltiazem	30 mg 4 times daily; titrate dose gradually at 1- to 2-d intervals; do not crush, cut, or chew
Verapamil	40 mg 3 times a d. May increase dose daily or weekly for max 480 mg/d

Data from Skidmore-Roth L. Mosby's drug guide for nursing students. 13th edition. St Louis (MO): Elsevier; 2019.

patients who exhibit life-threatening high-risk characteristics. High-risk characteristics include hemodynamic instability; cardiogenic shock; severe left ventricular dysfunction or heart failure; recurrent or persistent rest angina despite intensive medical therapy; new or worsening mitral regurgitation; new ventricular septal defect; and sustained ventricular arrhythmias.[8] Patient characteristics and risk factors help guide decisions regarding the urgency of invasive coronary revascularization.

Risk scores such as the Thrombolysis in Myocardial Infarction (TIMI) and Global Registry of Acute Coronary Events (GRACE) can be helpful for risk stratification of patients.[8] The TIMI risk score for ACS NSTEMI created by the *Thrombolysis in Myocardial Infarction Study Group* uses 7 variables to predict outcomes in patients with unstable angina or acute NSTEMI (**Table 6**).[16] Patients with higher TIMI scores (>3) gain more benefit from low-molecular-weight heparin, IIb/IIIa inhibitors, and an early invasive coronary intervention.

Another risk model used in the prediction of death and MI in hospital and at 6 months is the GRACE scoring system.[17] In hospital, admission at the time of the MI considers age, heart rate, systolic blood pressure, creatinine function, Killip heart failure classification, cardiac arrest on admission, ST-segment deviation, and elevation of cardiac biomarkers. Additional risk factors for 6-month predictions include in-hospital PCI, in-hospital coronary surgical revascularization, and past history of MI. An online calculator for the GRACE ACS Risk model can be found at http://www.outcomes-umassmed.org/grace/acs_risk/acs_risk_content.html. A GRACE score of greater than 140 is considered high-risk (**Table 7**).

Risk characteristics can help guide decisions regarding urgency of PCI (**Table 8**).[8] An early invasive intervention is indicated in patients considered to be at high risk, whereas patients with lower risk may benefit from a delayed invasive or ischemia-guided therapy.

Revascularization options for patients with NSTEMI include primary PCI and coronary artery bypass grafting (CABG).[8] Revascularization with PCI is performed most often, but CABG is the preferred option in patients with left main or left main equivalent disease, three- or two-vessel disease involving the left anterior descending artery with left ventricular dysfunction or diabetes.

Table 6 TIMI risk score	
Historical	
Age ≥65	+1
≥3 CAD risk factors	+1
Known CAD (stenosis ≥50%)	+1
ASA use in past 7 d	+1
Presentation	
Severe angina (≥2 episodes w/in 24 h)?	+1
+ Cardiac markers	+1
ST deviation ≥0.5 mm	+1

Abbreviation: CAD, coronary artery disease.

From TIMI Study Group. TIMI risk score calculator for UA/NSTEMI. Available at: http://www.timi.org/index.php?page=calculators. Accessed April 4, 2018; with permission.

Table 7
Risk of in-hospital death based on GRACE score

Risk Category	GRACE Risk Score	In-hospital Death (%)
Low	≤108	<1
Intermediate	109–140	1–3
High	>140	>3

From Global Registry of Acute Coronary Events. GRACE risk table. Available at: https://www.outcomes-umassmed.org/grace/grace_risk_table.aspx. Accessed October 19, 2018; with permission.

Adjunctive Therapy with Postpercutaneous Coronary Intervention for Non-ST-Elevation Myocardial Infarction

Antithrombotic therapy is recommended as an adjunct to primary PCI for NSTEMI.[12] Adjunctive antithrombotic therapy includes DAPT with both platelet inhibition and anticoagulation. Antiplatelet therapy consists of ASA and one of the P2Y$_{12}$ receptor inhibitors. ASA, 325 mg, should be given before PCI and continue indefinitely as a maintenance dose of 81 mg. P2Y$_{12}$ receptor inhibitor options include clopidogrel, prasugrel, or ticagrelor (see **Table 4**). A P2Y$_{12}$ loading dose should be administered as early as possible or at the time of PCI. A 1-year maintenance dose of a P2Y$_{12}$ inhibitor is recommended for all patients receiving a stent, bare metal, or drug eluding in the setting of NSTEMI. Unfractionated heparin, enoxaparin, fondaparinux or bivalirudin can be used for anticoagulant

Table 8
Strategy selection for patients with NSTEMI

Strategy	Risk Indicators
Immediate invasive (within 2 h)	Refractory angina Signs or symptoms of HF or new or worsening mitral regurgitation Hemodynamic instability Recurrent angina or ischemia at rest or with low-level activities despite intensive medical therapy Sustained VT or VF
Early invasive (within 24 h)	None of the abovementioned, but GRACE risk score >140 Temporal change in troponin New or presumably new ST depression
Delayed invasive (within 25–72 h)	None of the abovementioned but diabetes mellitus Renal insufficiency (GFR <60 mL/min/1.73 m^2) Reduced LV systolic function (EF <0.40) Early postinfarction angina PCI within 6 mo Prior coronary artery bypass grafting GRACE risk score of 109–140: TIMI score ≥2
Ischemia-guided strategy	Low-risk score (eg, TIMI [0 or 1], GRACE [109]) Low-risk troponin-negative female patients
	Patient or clinician preference in the absence of high-risk features

Abbreviations: EF, ejection fraction; GFR, glomerular filtration rate; HR, heart failure; LV, left ventricular; VF, ventricular fibrillation; VT, ventricular tachycardia.

From Amsterdam EA, Wenger NK, Brindis RG, et al. 2014 AHA/ACC guideline for the management of patients with non-ST-elevation acute coronary syndromes. J Am Coll Cardiol 2014;64:e168; with permission.

therapy. Intravenous IIb/IIIa inhibitors may be considered for initial antiplatelet therapy in high-risk patients receiving an early invasive strategy and those who have not had adequate pretreatment with one of the $P2Y_{12}$ inhibitors (**Table 9**).

ST-ELEVATION MYOCARDIAL INFARCTION

Early reperfusion therapy is the mainstay of treatment for patients presenting with an acute STEMI. Options for reperfusion therapy include primary PCI, fibrinolytic therapy, or urgent CABG. Generally, primary PCI is the recommended reperfusion strategy when available within the recommended time window and the coronary anatomy is amenable to PCI.[12] Delays to reperfusion therapy have been associated with high mortality rates. Because of the time sensitive nature of therapy, appropriate and timely reperfusion is more important than the form of reperfusion therapy. It is critical for emergency departments to have protocols and processes in place to facilitate prompt recognition and treatment of patients presenting with STEMI.

Initial Therapy

PCI of the culprit artery is the preferred reperfusion strategy for patients presenting with STEMI and symptom onset within the prior 12 hours.[12] Timely PCI has been associated with reduced mortality and lowered rates of recurrent ischemia and MACE. The goal for first medical contact (FMC)-to-device (balloon ± stent) time is 90 minutes or less. When patients present to a non-PCI capable hospital, transfer to a PCI-capable hospital is recommended if FMC-to-device time can be achieved in 120 minutes or less. If timely transfer to a PCI-capable hospital is not possible, the preferred reperfusion strategy is fibrinolytic therapy. For patients presenting with STEMI and symptom onset within the prior 12 to 24 hours, PCI is preferred over fibrinolytic therapy, but if PCI is not available and there are no absolute contraindications, fibrinolytic therapy is recommended over no reperfusion therapy.

Nonculprit Vessels

Multivessel coronary disease is found in approximately 50% of patients presenting with STEMI.[18] Addressing disease of nonculprit vessels with PCI at the time of early

Table 9 IIb/IIIa inhibitors				
IIb/IIIa Inhibitor	Loading Dose	Infusion Dose	Duration	Other
Abciximab	0.25 mg/kg	0.125 mcg/kg/min (max 10 mcg/min)	18–24 h	Not recommended if catheterization is delayed for more than 4 h
Eptifibatide	180 mcg/kg (max 22.6 mg) Repeat 180 mcg/kg bolus in 10 min	2 mcg/kg/min (max 15 mg/h)	18–24 h	Creatinine clearance <50 mL/min—reduce infusion dose by 50%
Tirofiban	25 mcg/kg	0.15 mcg/kg/min	Up to 18 h	Creatinine clearance <60 mL/min—reduce infusion dose by 50%

Data from Gahart BL, Nazareno AR, Ortega MQ. Intravenous medications: a handbook for nurses and health professionals. 35th edition. St Louis (MO): Elsevier; 2019.

invasive intervention is not recommended in hemodynamically unstable patients unless high-risk findings are present. PCI intervention for noninfarct artery vessels in hemodynamically unstable patients should be planned and staged later when hemodynamic stability has been achieved. It is reasonable to consider noninfarct artery PCI at the time of culprit artery PCI in hemodynamically stable patients.

Adjunctive Therapy with Postpercutaneous Coronary Intervention for ST-Elevation Myocardial Infarction

Antithrombotic therapy is recommended as an adjunct to primary PCI for STEMI. Adjunctive antithrombotic therapy includes DAPT with both platelet inhibition and anticoagulation. DAPT consists of ASA and one of the $P2Y_{12}$ receptor inhibitors.[12] DAPT for STEMI follows the same guidelines as recommend in the NSTEMI adjunctive therapy with PCI section.

Antiplatelet therapy using intravenous glycoprotein (GP) IIb/IIIa receptor antagonists are not routinely used with PCI for STEMI but could be considered in patients who have a large thrombus burden or inadequate $P2Y_{12}$ receptor inhibitor loading. Options for intravenous GP IIb/IIIa receptor antagonist include abciximab, high bolus dose tirofiban, or double-bolus eptifibatide (see **Table 9**).

Patients treated with primary PCI for STEMI should receive anticoagulant therapy at the time of the intervention. Bolus dosing of unfractionated heparin to maintain therapeutic activated clotting time levels or bivalirudin are both recommended options for primary PCI with STEMI (**Table 10**).

In summary, adjunctive antithrombotic therapy for STEMI includes antiplatelet and anticoagulation therapy. Anticoagulant therapy is administered at the time of PCI. Dual antiplatelet therapy is administered as soon as possible with loading and maintenance doses. Maintenance dosing of ASA is continued indefinitely and maintenance dosing of $P2Y_{12}$ receptor inhibitors are continued for 1 year.

Fibrinolytic Therapy

For patients with STEMI presenting to a non-PCI capable hospital, fibrinolytic therapy is recommended when symptom onset is within the prior 12 hours, and transfer to a PCI-capable hospital cannot be achieved within the recommended time window (FMC-to-device $\leq$120 minutes).[12] Before administration of any fibrinolytic therapy, patients must be evaluated for eligibility, ruling out any contraindications and weighing the potential benefit versus risk (**Box 4**). The benefit of fibrinolytic therapy rapidly declines 3 hours after onset of symptoms. When fibrinolytic therapy is the chosen reperfusion strategy, the goal to administration time is 30 minutes from diagnosis of STEMI. When symptom onset is within the prior 12 to 24 hours and patients exhibit ongoing clinical and/or ECG evidence of ongoing ischemia, fibrinolytic therapy is considered reasonable but primary PCI is the preferred strategy.

Table 10 Anticoagulant therapy for PCI with STEMI	
Anticoagulant	**Notes**
Unfractionated heparin (UFH)	Bolus dosing to maintain therapeutic activated clotting time levels
Bivalirudin	With or without prior treatment with UFH

Data from O'Gara PT, Kushner FG, Ascheim DD, et al. 2013 ACCF/AHA guideline for the management of ST-elevation myocardial infarction. Circulation 2013;127:E362–425.

Box 4
Contraindications to fibrinolytic therapy

Absolute Contraindications

- A prior intracranial hemorrhage
- Known structural cerebral vascular lesion (eg, arteriovenous malformation)
- Known malignant intracranial neoplasm (primary or metastatic)
- Ischemic stroke within 3 months EXCEPT acute ischemic stroke within 3 hours
- Suspected aortic dissection
- Active bleeding or bleeding diathesis (excluding menses)
- Significant closed head trauma or facial trauma within 3 months

Relative Contraindications

- History of chronic, severe, poorly controlled hypertension
- Severe uncontrolled hypertension on presentation (SBP >180 mm Hg or >110 mm Hg)
- History of prior ischemic stroke >3 months, dementia, or known intracranial pathology not covered in contraindications.
- Traumatic or prolonged (>10 minutes) CPR or major surgery (<3 weeks)
- Recent (within 2–4 weeks) internal bleeding
- Noncompressible vascular punctures
- For streptokinase/anistreplase: prior exposure (>5 days ago) or prior allergic reaction to these agents
- Pregnancy
- Active peptic ulcer
- Current use of anticoagulants: the higher the INR, the higher the risk of bleeding

Abbreviations: CPR, cardiopulmonary resuscitation; INR, international normalized ratio; SBP, systolic blood pressure.
Data from American Heart Association. Advanced cardiac life support provider manual. Dallas (TX): American Heart Association; 2016.

Fibrinolytic options available for use with STEMI patients include the fibrin-specific agents tenecteplase, reteplase, and alteplase and the nonfibrin-specific agent, streptokinase.[8] When available, fibrin-specific agents are preferred over the nonfibrin-specific agents. Fibrin specific agents include tenecteplase, reteplase and alteplase, and streptokinase is a non-fibrin specific agent.[12] The decision to use fibrinolytic therapy in patients with STEMI is made based on a risk-benefit analysis guided by the absolute and relative contraindications to fibrinolytic therapy and other patient characteristics. Characteristics that inform the decision include time of symptom onset, clinical and hemodynamic features at presentation, patient comorbidities, risk of bleeding, presence of contraindications, and time delay to PCI. After fibrinolysis is complete, arrangements for transfer to a PCI-capable hospital for early coronary angiography and possible PCI is recommended.

A plan for early transfer to a PCI-capable hospital for coronary angiography and evaluation for revascularization should be established for patients receiving fibrinolytic therapy.[12] Immediate transfer to a PCI-capable hospital is recommended for all patients who develop cardiogenic shock or acute severe heart failure. Urgent transfer is recommended for failed reperfusion or reocclusion after fibrinolytic therapy.

Table 11 Anticoagulant therapy with fibrinolysis	
Anticoagulant	**Dose**
Unfractionated heparin	Weight-based bolus plus infusion titrated to achieve a partial thromboplastin time of 1.5–2 times control
Enoxaparin	Dose according to age, weight, and creatinine clearance given IV followed by SQ injection
Fondaparinux	Initial IV dose followed in 24 h by daily SQ if creatinine clearance is >30 mL/min

Abbreviations: IV, intravenous; SQ, subcutaneous.
Data from Amsterdam EA, Wenger NK, Brindis RG, et al. 2014 AHA/ACC guideline for the management of patients with non-ST-elevation acute coronary syndromes. J Am Coll Cardiol 2014;64:e139–228.

Transfer of stable patients with successful fibrinolysis is recommended when logistically feasible, ideally within 24 hours but not within the first 2 to 3 hours after administration of fibrinolytic therapy.

Anticoagulant Therapy with Fibrinolysis

Anticoagulant therapy is recommended for patients receiving fibrinolysis for NSTEMI.[8] Anticoagulant regimens include unfractionated heparin, intravenous enoxaparin or fondaparinux (**Table 11**). Therapy is recommended for a minimum of 48 hours and preferably for the duration of hospitalization (up to 8 days) or until revascularization is complete.

Emergent Coronary Aartery Bypass Grafting

Except for cases of cardiogenic shock, CABG is not a first-line strategy for patients presenting with STEMI.[12] Situations where CABG might be indicated include failed PCI, when coronary anatomy is not amenable to PCI, or urgent surgical repair is indicated for mechanical defects such as ventricular septal, papillary muscle, or free-wall rupture. Mechanical circulatory support devices (ie, ventricular assist devices) may be indicated as an adjunct for hemodynamically unstable patients in need of urgent CABG. Use of off-pump surgical techniques and mechanical circulatory support devices may lead to improved survival rates.

PREVENTION

Focus of this article has largely been on recognition and management of NSTEMI/STEMI; however, prevention should play a primary role in practice. Prevention of CAD focuses on strategies that improve cardiovascular health.[2] The AHA "Life's Simple 7" campaign provides patients and providers with 7 health indicators to prevent CAD[2]: blood pressure, physical activity, cholesterol, diet, weight, tobacco use, and blood glucose levels.[2] Maintaining cardiovascular health by focusing on these 7 health indicators is associated with a lower risk of cardiovascular disease, cardiovascular mortality, and all-cause mortality.[2]

SUMMARY

Although incidence of MI has demonstrated a significant decline over the past few years, Americans still experience 790,000 MIs annually.[2] Early recognition, appropriate diagnosis, and proper management of patients presenting with NSTEMI/STEMI are imperative to ensuring improved patient outcomes in the hospital and after discharge. Standard medical therapy for any patient presenting with suspected NSTEMI/STEMI includes oxygen therapy when appropriate, nitrate administration unless contraindicated, analgesic therapy with morphine, administration of beta-adrenergic blockers within 24 hours, and antiplatelet therapy with ASA and a $P2Y_{12}$ inhibitor.[8] CCBs may also be considered in patients with intractable angina who have received optimal treatment with beta-blockers.[8] In addition, high-intensity statin therapy is recommended for all patients with NSTEMI/STEMI.[8]

Management of NSTEMI includes ischemia-guided therapy or medical management. Invasive coronary intervention is not recommended unless the patient presents with life-threatening high-risk characteristics (see **Table 8**).[8] In STEMI, early reperfusion therapy with PCI is the mainstay of therapy.[12] Fibrinolytic therapy may be the preferred reperfusion therapy for STEMI in non-PCI capable facilities where FMC-to-device cannot be achieved within the recommended time window of 120 minutes.[12] CABG is only considered a first-line strategy for STEMI in cases of cardiogenic shock.[12]

Finally, prevention of coronary artery disease resulting NSTEMI/STEMI should play a large part in practice. Optimal blood pressure, physical activity, cholesterol, diet, weight, tobacco use, and blood glucose levels are associated with lower risk of cardiovascular disease and a decline in the NSTEMI/STEMI.[2]

REFERENCES

1. National Center for Health Statistics. Health, United States, 2015: with special feature in racial and ethnic health disparities. Centers for Disease Control and Prevention. Available at: https://www.cdc.gov/nchs/data/hus/hus15.pdf. Accessed May 3, 2018.

2. Benjamin EJ, Blaha MJ, Chiuve SE, et al. Heart disease and stroke statistics—2017 update: a report from the American Heart Association. Circulation 2017; 135(10). https://doi.org/10.1161/cir.0000000000000485.

3. Ford ES, Roger VL, Dunlay SM, et al. Challenges of ascertaining national trends in the incidence of coronary heart disease in the United States. J Am Heart Assoc 2014;3(6):e001097.

4. Boudi FB. Risk factors for coronary artery disease. In: Subhi Y, editor. MedScape. Available at: https://emedicine.medscape.com/article/164163-overview. Accessed May 3, 2018.

5. Reigle J. Coronary circulation disorders. In: Sorenson M, Quinn L, Klein D, editors. Pathophysiology: concepts of human disease. Hoboken (NJ): Pearson; 2019. p. 572–611.

6. Mann DL, Zipes DP, Libby P, et al. Braunwald's heart disease: a textbook of cardiovascular medicine. 10th edition. Philadelphia: Elsevier; 2015.

7. Zafari AM. Myocardial infarction workup. In Yang EH, editor. MedScape. Available at: https://emedicine.medscape.com/article/155919-workup. Accessed May 3, 2018.

8. Amsterdam EA, Wenger NK, Brindis RG, et al. 2014 AHA/ACC guideline for the management of patients with non-ST-elevation acute coronary syndromes. J Am Coll Cardiol 2014;64:e139–228.

9. Ellis KM. Myocardial infarction. In: EKG plain and simple. 4th edition. Boston: Pearson Education; 2016. p. 311–43.

10. Thygesen K, Alpert JS, Jaffe AS, et al. Third universal definition of myocardial infarction. J Am Coll Cardiol 2012;60(16):1581–98.

11. McCarthy CP, Donnellan E, Wasfy JG, et al. Time-honored treatments for the initial management of acute coronary syndromes: challenging the status quo. Trends Cardiovasc Med 2017;27:483–91. Available at: https://www.sciencedirect.com/science/article/pii/S1050173817300555?via%3Dihub. Accessed February 20, 2018.

12. O'Gara PT, Kushner FG, Ascheim DD, et al. 2013 ACCF/AHA guideline for the management of ST-elevation myocardial infarction. Circulation 2013;127: E362–425. Available at: https://www.heart.org/idc/groups/heart-public/@wcm/@mwa/documents/downloadable/ucm_458913.pdf. Accessed February 28, 2018.

13. Maalouf R, Mosley M, Kallail J, et al. A comparison of salicylic acid levels in normal subjects after rectal versus oral dosing. Acad Emerg Med 2009;16(2): 157–61.

14. Levine GN, Bates ER, Bittl JA, et al. 2016 ACC/AHA guideline focused update on duration of dual antiplatelet therapy in patients with coronary artery disease. J Am Coll Cardiol 2016;68:1082–115.

15. Stone NJ, Robinson J, Lichtenstein AH, et al. 2013 ACC/AHA Guideline on the treatment of blood cholesterol to reduce atherosclerotic cardiovascular risk in adults. Circulation 2014;129(25 Suppl 2):S1–45.

16. TIMI Risk Score Calculator for UA/NSTEMI. TIMI Study Group. Available at: http://www.timi.org/index.php?page=calculators. Accessed April 4, 2018.

17. ACS Risk Score: Risk Stratification. Global Registry of Acute Coronary Events. http://gracescore.co.uk/risk-stratification. Available at: Accessed May 25, 2018.

18. Levine GN, Bates ER, Blankenship JC, et al. 2016 ACC/AHA/SCAI Focused update on primary percutaneous intervention for patients with ST-elevation myocardial infarction. J Am Coll Cardiol 2016;67(10):1235–50.

Nursing Management for Patients Postoperative Cardiac Implantable Electronic Device Placement

Leanne H. Fowler, DNP, MBA, APRN, AGACNP-BC, CNE

KEYWORDS

- Critical care • ICU • Nurse • Implanted cardiac device

KEY POINTS

- The number of implantable cardiac devices used as therapeutic options are steadily increasing.
- Adults 70 years and older are the most common population using implantable cardiac devices.
- Critical care nurses can improve postoperative patient outcomes when applying knowledge to patient care.

The number of individuals with cardiac implantable electronic devices (CIEDs) has increased over the past 10 to 20 years.[1] CIEDs include permanent pacemakers (PPMs), implanted cardioverter-defibrillators (ICDs), cardiac resynchronization therapy (CRT), implantable loop recorders, and implantable cardiovascular monitors.[2] Individuals undergoing the procedure for implantation require clinicians with the fundamental knowledge of indications warranting CIEDs, the surgical approach for implantation, the therapeutic effects, and the complications associated with the surgical procedure and with long-term implantation of the device. This knowledge will support nurses with the skills needed for the postoperative management of CIED patients and with the information to provide comprehensive patient education. The scope of this article is limited to the knowledge critical care nurses can apply to patients with PPMs, ICDs, and CRT. Implanted cardiac event recorders are not discussed.

EPIDEMIOLOGY

Epidemiologic data regarding CIEDs are difficult to obtain due to differences in reporting procedures between inpatient and outpatient clinical agencies. The data reported

Disclosure Statement: The author has nothing to disclose.
LSU Health New Orleans School of Nursing, 1900 Gravier Street, New Orleans, LA 70112, USA
E-mail address: lfowle@lsuhsc.edu

by inpatient agencies demonstrate men between 64 to 84 years of age have the highest incidence for CIED placement, PPMs and ICDs alike. Additionally, cardiac device–related complication rates are lower for single chamber devices versus dual-chamber devices but are higher among adults 70 years and older who have any CIED with lead placement.[3] CIED placement is proven to prolong life and the quality of life.[2] However, in individuals with progressive cardiac disease and individuals with noncardiac comorbidities (eg, diabetes mellitus, chronic kidney disease, chronic liver disease,), implanted cardiac devices can pose complications that increase morbidity and mortality rates. The complication with the highest mortality rate is CIED-related infection.[1,3]

CARDIAC IMPLANTED ELECTRONIC DEVICES

The devices discussed in this article have similar and unique characteristics and functionality. PPMs are discussed in greater depth than ICDs, CRT, or cardiovascular monitors owing to the many similarities in functionality. Device-specific sections primarily discuss unique characteristics not already discussed.

Permanent pacemaker

Cardiac pacemakers were first introduced to cardiac disease management in the 1950s. There are external and internal pacemakers, and temporary pacemakers and PPMs. Conventional PPMs are internal and consist of an implanted battery-powered electrical pulse generator connected to pacing leads embedded into the endocardium. Since inception, PPMs have evolved in size, battery life, and its use of leads. Likewise, since inception, the surgical approach for PPM placement and associated complications have also evolved to safer practices and improved patient outcomes.[4] Today, leadless PPMs are available and have been approved by the US Federal Food and Drug Administration. Leadless PPMs offer a nonsurgical approach and fewer lead-related complications.[5]

Indications

PPMs are most often used to treat or to prevent cardiac arrhythmias. Arrhythmias indicating the need for PPM placement include sinus and/or atrioventricular node dysfunction, heart blocks secondary to neuromuscular disorders, atrial fibrillation, documented periods of asystole, and medical therapies resulting in bradycardia.[2,6] Other indications warranting PPM placement include cardiac transplantation, neuromuscular diseases, sleep apnea syndrome, cardiac sarcoidosis, congenital heart disease, and for hemodynamic alterations. PPMs are also indicated for the prevention or termination of arrhythmias such as atrial fibrillation, other atrial arrhythmias, and long QT syndrome.[2,6] Leadless PPMs have fewer indications but are similar (**Table 1**).

Contraindications associated with conventional PPM are fewer than its leadless PPM counterpart. Conventional PPMs (transvenous placement of leads) are absolutely contraindicated for a patient with a mechanical atrioventricular valve. An epicardial PPM is warranted for this patient. Other contraindications include active infections and hemodynamic instability.[2,6] Leadless PPMs are contraindicated for patients with implanted vena cava filters, mechanical tricuspid valves, or implanted cardiac devices providing active therapy.[7]

Ongoing research is being conducted to identify the utility of PPMs in the setting of individuals with advanced heart failure who are in need of left ventricular assist devices (LVADs). To date, there are limited data demonstrating the safe and tolerable use of PPMs or any CIEDs concurrently with LVADs for an already vulnerable population.[8]

Table 1
Indications for permanent pacemaker placement

Conventional PPM	Leadless PPM
• Sinus node dysfunction • Acquired AV block in adults • Chronic fascicular block • AV block after AMI • Hypersensitive carotid sinus syndrome and neurocardiogenic syncope • Cardiac transplantation • Neuromuscular diseases • Sleep apnea syndrome • Cardiac sarcoidosis • Prevention of atrial arrhythmias or long QT syndrome • Obstructive HCM • Congenital heart disease	• Sinus node dysfunction when atrial or dual chamber pacing is high risk • Symptomatic paroxysmal or permanent high-grade AV block in the presence of AF ○ In the absence of AF when dual chamber is high risk

Abbreviations: AF, atrial fibrillation; AMI, acute myocardial infarction; AV, atrioventricular; HCM, hypertrophic cardiomyopathy.

Mechanism of Action

A conventional PPM pulse generator emits electricity to the heart through electrical leads within the desired heart chamber (atria, ventricular, or both). These devices are more complex than temporary pacemakers owing to their diverse functional offerings and ability for numerous settings. PPM settings are individualized to meet the electrophysiological needs of each patient.

Conventional PPM devices can sense bradyarrhythmias or tachyarrhythmias. Bradyarrhythmias can be sensed below a set threshold and paced to a higher prescribed rate as desired. The prescribed rate can be set to deliver impulses when needed (ie, inhibited or demand pacing) or permanently to prevent the heart's intrinsic rate being lower than desired. Tachyarrhythmias can also be sensed and overdrive-paced to capture and lower the patient's intrinsic rate. The pacemaker technologist or interventional cardiologist sets the PPM impulses.[4]

Leadless PPMs are the latest evolved devices that aim to perform many of the same functions as the conventional PPM but without transvenous leads. These devices are fully self-contained with a pulse generator, battery, and electrodes within an encapsulated unit comparatively measuring close to 1 cm^3. The specific size of the leadless PPM is 42 mm in length and 5.99 mm in diameter.[5]

Device settings

The complexity of PPM functionality involves its variety of settings. Although complex, this variety allows the interventional cardiologist or electrophysiologist to customize its function to each patient. A revised generic code for pacemaker settings designed in 2002 by the North American Society of Pacing and Electrophysiology (NASPE) and the British Pacing and Electrophysiology Group (BPEG) is still being used. The revised code is aimed to improve the standardization of the language used for pacing and to eliminate confusion by enhancing communication among all health care providers (**Table 2**).[9]

The revised code has 5 positions. Positions I through III indicate the chambers being sensed and paced. Sensing is defined as the device's ability to detect an individual's intrinsic cardiac depolarization. Pacing refers to the device's pulse generator emitting electricity into the heart muscle to cause depolarization.[9]

Table 2 Revised North American Society of Pacing and Electrophysiology and the British Pacing and Electrophysiology Group pacing code				
I	II	III	VI	V
Chamber Paced	Chamber Sensed	Response to Sensing	Rate Modulation	Multisite Pacing
O = None	O = None	O = None	O = None	O = None
A = Atria	A = Atria	T = Triggered	R = Adaptive rate	A = Atria
V = Ventricle	V = Ventricle	I = Inhibited		V = Ventricle
D = Dual	D = Dual	D = Dual		D = Dual

Adapted from Bernstein AD, Daubert J-C, Fletcher RD, et al. The revised NASPE/BPEG generic code for antibradycardia, adaptive-rate, and multisite pacing. Pacing Clin Electrophysiol 2002;25(2):261; with permission.

Position IV in the generic pacing code indicates the device having (denoted as R) or not having (denoted as O) the adaptive rate, or rate modulation, function. The adaptive rate function allows the device to provide a rate higher than the lowest set rate in response to the individual's activity level. Position V in the generic pacing code indicates whether pacing is present in both atria, both ventricles, or in all 4 chambers.[9]

Nurses should have a basic understanding of the NASPE-BPEG pacing code to understand the actions the device takes for their patient. For example, a patient with a generic pacing code of DDDOV has a dual-chambered PPM with the function of dual-chamber, biventricular pacing (D in position I, V in position V), dual-chamber sensing with a triggered and inhibitory function (D in positions II and III), and no adaptive-rate mechanism (O in position IV).

Therapeutic effects

The primary and intended effects of PPMs are to help stabilize cardiac arrhythmias, improve hemodynamic stability, and improve cardiac function.[2] Rate-response mechanisms improve the patients' symptoms caused by sinus node dysfunction (chronotropic incompetence) during activities of daily living. In patients with second-degree and third-degree atrioventricular blocks, PPMs prevent associated syncope and bradyarrhythmias. Additionally, PPMs improve survival rates in individuals with third-degree atrioventricular blocks.[6] Despite the many therapeutic effects PPMs offer patients, pharmacotherapeutic agents may still be needed in adjunct to device therapy to achieve the patient's desired state.

Indirect or unintended effects of individuals having PPMs include the device documenting asymptomatic periods of atrial fibrillation. Asymptomatic periods of atrial fibrillation or other subclinical tachyarrhythmias are defined as an atrial rate greater than or equal to 190 beats per minute lasting greater than or equal to 6 minutes. Subclinical tachyarrhythmia events place the patient at a 2.5-fold increased risk for ischemic stroke or systemic embolism. Subclinical, device-documented atrial fibrillation places the patient at a 4-fold to 5-fold risk for stroke within the initial 5 to 10 days of the episode.[3]

Surgical approach

An interventional cardiologist in an inpatient cardiac suite or cardiac catheter laboratory most often performs the placement of conventional PPMs. However, electrophysiologists can also place these devices, which can occur within an office-like setting or an electrophysiology laboratory. Conventional PPM placement is considered a surgical procedure. The patient is administered a penicillin-based prophylactic antimicrobial and the skin is scrubbed with bactericidal and antiseptic preparation before incision. The skin is incised to make a pouch within the upper left or upper right chest wall just below the clavicles via a cut-down technique. The cut-down technique allows the cardiac specialist to create a pocket within the subcutaneous tissue to house the pulse generator, and to visualize and access the subclavian, axillary, or cephalic vein for lead cannulation and placement within the endocardium. After leads placement is verified to be in the desired chamber by fluoroscopy, they are then connected to the pulse generator for testing. When testing is complete and the device is verified to be functioning as desired, the pulse generator is placed within the chest wall pocket and the skin is closed with sutures and secured with antimicrobial dressing aimed to prevent postoperative infection.[4,10]

Placement of the leadless PPM takes a nonsurgical, percutaneous approach for placement. An interventional cardiologist delivers the device with a catheter cannulating the femoral vein to the right ventricle for implantation. The device is then embedded or implanted directly into the muscle of the right ventricle and eliminates the need to create a chest wall pocket, cannulation of the subclavian vein with rigid leads, and repeatedly flexing the cardiac lead for the purpose of muscle implantation, which can cause lead damage with these mechanics during each heartbeat.[5]

Complications

The adverse events related to PPMs are most often due to the transvenous leads, a surgical pocket within the chest wall, or the pulse generator. PPM leads can be dislodged, can fracture, and can undergo insulation failure, leading to venous occlusion, cardiac perforation, tricuspid valve dysfunction, and infection. Pulse generators placed into a surgically created chest wall pocket are at risk for infection, skin erosion, or bleeding that can cause a hematoma.[11,12]

Leadless PPMs eliminate the risk of chest wall pocket, lead, and tricuspid valve complications. However, complications occurring with the leadless device include[5] possible complications with the leadless device, including allergic reaction, oversensing, exacerbating tachycardia, myocardial infarction, and those associated with placement of the device (ie, cardiac perforation, pericardial effusion, cardiac tamponade, and device embolization).[7]

Twiddler syndrome

Overmanipulation of the pulse generator by twisting or rotating it within the pocket is known as Twiddler syndrome. Affected patients often inadvertently dislodge or damage the CIED leads and cause device malfunction. Patients often present urgently or emergently due to symptomatic bradycardia, particularly if they are pacemaker-dependent.

Infections

Increasing rates of conventional CIED infections are multifactorial. Conventional PPMs and ICDs (see later discussion) have similar susceptibility to CIED-associated infections. Considering the widespread use of broad-spectrum antibiotics, varying prophylactic measures, and changing patient demographics and characteristics, infection rates associated with CIED leads, the device, and the pocket are increasing.[13] For instance, CIED recipients are increasingly older (>70–80 years old) and have multiple comorbidities. These patients have higher needs, not only for the increased use of devices aimed to reduce morbidity and mortality but also for added hardware (eg, dual-chamber pacing, biventricular pacing). Increased hardware burden places the older adult with multiple comorbidities at risk for all CIED-associated complications but particularly endovascular, endocardial, and device or pocket infections.[13]

When device leads malfunction, the practice of disconnecting, capping, and leaving the lead or leads embedded in the endocardium but disconnected from the pulse generator is thought to be the leading cause in the increase of device infections. However, extracting CIED leads poses risks for perforation, myocardial rupture, and embolism of lead vegetation. Lead extraction is risky but sometimes necessary to eradicate CIED-associated infections and ultimately reduce the patient's morbidity and mortality.[1]

After extraction of CIEDs (leads and generator), the risk for cardiac device–related infective endocarditis persists. This risk is thought to be associated with floating intracardiac masses (also known as ghosts) found by echocardiography after device removal. The presence of ghosts was found in known infected patients who were diagnosed with infective endocarditis using blood cultures. Ghosts were not found in noninfected patients after device removal.[14]

Device (orthopedic or cardiac) infections pose a unique risk to patients due to the most commonly associated microorganisms' ability to resist antimicrobials. CIED-associated infections increase the patient's risk for increased morbidity and mortality owing to its nature for endovascular implantation and automatic exposure of the microorganisms to the bloodstream. The leading cause of conventional CIED-associated infections involves the staphylococcal species, both methicillin-sensitive microbes and methicillin-resistant microbes.[13] Staphylococcal species are most often acquired from health care environments and have an ability to develop a biofilm around themselves. A biofilm facilitates the microbe's adhesion to devices and protects it from the bactericidal or bacteriostatic effects of most antibiotics.[15] A patient's frequent exposure to hospital or health care environments, age, comorbidities, and implantation with a cardiac device poses a unique risk and vulnerability of patients that nurses must recognize.

Electromagnetic interference
External sources of electromagnetic currents can cause PPM inference with accurately sensing the patient's intrinsic electricity and can thereby also interfere with pacing accuracy. Cellular telephones, surveillance systems, magnets, and welding equipment are all potential sources of electromagnetic interference.[16] Patients can also experience electromagnetic interference when undergoing surgical or invasive procedures using electrocautery, radio frequencies, radiation, or magnets.[17]

Implanted Cardioverter-Defibrillator
The ICD was introduced as a therapeutic device in the 1980s. The device is difficult to differentiate from a conventional PPM except in its larger size of the pulse generator and a single-chamber lead able to sense and shock life-threatening ventricular arrhythmias.[4] The ICDs, like the PPM, has evolved in functionality to now have dual functions as both a pacemaker and cardioverter-defibrillator.[10]

Indications
Formerly, the primary indication for ICD placement was for patients who survived cardiac arrest and failed antiarrhythmic pharmacotherapy. With continued research, indications have broadened to include ICD therapy as primary and secondary prophylactic measures for sudden cardiac death, cardiac arrest, and sustained ventricular tachycardia. Individuals with dilated or ischemic cardiomyopathies, with recent (<48–72 hours) acute myocardial infarction, and with heart failure with reduced ejection fraction (HFrEF) (<40%–45%) are at the greatest risk for recurrent, sustained ventricular tachycardia and/or ventricular fibrillation. The high risk for lethal ventricular

arrhythmias is the primary indication for ICD placements aimed to reduce morbidity and mortality rates among affected patients in whom pharmacotherapy has been proven not to be effective.[6]

Contraindications for ICD placement include any ventricular tachyarrhythmias that are reversible (eg, drug toxicity, trauma, and electrolyte imbalance) and are not associated with structural abnormalities, tachyarrhythmias in patients in whom other therapies should be considered first (eg, pharmacotherapy, catheter ablation), and for patients with active infections and/or hemodynamic instability.[18]

Mechanism of action
The sensing and pacing mechanisms within the ICD device work to sense and pace the heart as needed, similar to the demand mechanisms of a PPM. In addition to the cardioverter-defibrillator lead within the device, additional pacing leads can be placed in other heart chambers for dual-chamber and multisite functionality, as in the PPM device.

Functioning of the cardioverter-defibrillator lead requires contact with a larger surface area than a PPM lead. Therefore, this lead is designed as a coiled wire intended to embed within a larger port of the ventricular myocardium than a pacing lead would. Nevertheless, the cardioverter-defibrillator lead is able to execute PPM and ICD functions.

Therapeutic effects
The therapeutic effects for ICD therapy includes those afforded by PPMs. In addition to the benefits of PPM, an ICD primarily reduces the patient's morbidity and mortality rates related to lethal ventricular arrhythmias and sudden cardiac death.[6,8] Primary prophylactic use of ICD therapy for patients with HFrEF remains debatable owing to varying research study results nationally and varying reported practices among cardiologists.[19] Early termination of ventricular tachycardia and ventricular fibrillation by ICD therapy has reduced the mortality rate for sudden cardiac death.[3,6]

Surgical approach
The surgical approach to ICD placement is the same approach used for PPM placement. However, as previously mentioned, the cardioverter-defibrillator lead placement is implanted within the ventricle's myocardium, whereas only the PPM lead tip is embedded into the endocardium.[1]

Complications
The complications associated with ICD devices are inclusive of those associated with PPMs. Complications specific to ICD devices are associated with the inappropriate delivery of shocks and any adverse (unintended) effects experienced by appropriate shocks. Lead fractures and impaired sensing can cause inappropriate shock delivery. Adverse effects of appropriate shocks delivered to patients can cause anxiety, restrict individuals from driving, and can negatively affect the patient's quality of life.[20] Electromagnetic interference specifically with ICD devices can occur with the electrocauterization equipment used in surgery.[16]

Cardiac resynchronization therapy
Multisite ventricular pacing is also known as CRT or biventricular pacing. CRT uses a pulse generator and electrical leads as the PPM and ICD devices do. Functionality differs in which the CRT device delivers impulses to bilateral chambers (ie, both ventricles) in an effort to resynchronize the electrical and mechanical work of the heart for patients with HFrEF, cardiac remodeling, and arrhythmias causing dyssynchrony. Such resynchronization supports hemodynamic stability and improves ventricular

ejection fraction for patients with HFrEF. The evolution of CRT includes the device's functionality to include CRT-defibrillation (CRT-D). Therefore, patients with dyssynchrony who are at risk for sustained ventricular tachycardia, recurrent syncope, or sudden cardiac death gain the therapeutic effects of ICD therapy.[2]

Indications
CRT is primarily indicated in patients with HFrEF less than 30% to 35% and symptomatic cardiac dyssynchrony caused prolonged QRS greater than 150 milliseconds (class I recommendation) who are already receiving maximal goal-directed pharmacotherapy. CRT is not recommended for patients whose frailty and comorbidities limits their lifespan to less than 1 year because studies did not show any provided benefit (class III recommendation).[2] Contraindications for CRT mirror those for PPMs and ICDs.

Therapeutic effect
CRT modifies ventricular electromechanical delay through multisite or biventricular pacing. This therapy provides select HFrEF patients improved hemodynamic stability and improved quality of life by reducing symptoms of dyspnea on exertion, chest tightness, palpitations, and syncope. CRT-D improves mortality rates for HFrEF patients at risk for sudden cardiac death.[2,21]

POSTOPERATIVE MANAGEMENT

The critical care nurses can often be the clinicians caring for a patient immediately status post-CIED placement. Knowledge and skills for immediate postoperative management are necessary for the early detection of device dysfunction, infection control, and patient and/or family education. Knowledge and skills associated with long-term postoperative CIED management are also necessary for critical care nurses when critically ill patients also have CIEDs in situ. The fundamental critical care knowledge needed for postoperative management that is not discussed includes electrocardiogram interpretation and analysis, hemodynamic alterations analysis and management, and pharmacotherapeutic knowledge.

Patient Assessment

Immediate postoperative cardiac implantable electronic device placement
Critical care nurses should have an understanding of the underlying disease process of the patient, the type of CIED placed, the therapeutic effects, and potential complications. For instance, patients who underwent single- chamber conventional PPM placement should be on a cardiac monitor to assess for pacing capture, for hemodynamic stability, and for arrhythmias that persist. A review of systems and physical examination should be conducted regularly (per patient acuity and specialist orders) to evaluate the patient for complaints and adverse effects or events. For instance, a patient complaining of palpitations status post-PPM placement may have sensed the device overdrive pacing a tachyarrhythmia. Interrogation of the device is needed to confirm. Critical care nurses now have access to point-of-care interrogation devices to facilitate point-of-care decisions and communication with the cardiologist or other specialists.

Patients undergoing CIED placement or repair can have anticoagulants among their list of home medications. There are growing data to support the safe uninterrupted use of non–vitamin K antagonists during CIED implantation.[22] Critical care nurses should monitor for postoperative bleeding and a pocket hematoma in all patients but particularly patients who have chronic anticoagulation for stroke or other thrombotic risk reduction.

Long-term postoperative cardiac implantable electronic device management

Patients with CIEDs in situ should be assessed for signs and symptoms of infection, hemodynamic stability, and device malfunction. Individuals with CIEDs in situ admitted to the critical care unit with bloodstream infections are vulnerable to the devices becoming infected. Critical care nurses must facilitate the timely treatment of infections in these patients by ensuring the appropriate collection of blood cultures, avoiding delays in antimicrobial treatment, using prudent universal precautions and aseptic techniques with the manipulation of invasive lines and drains, and using skillful communication with the health care team. For patients undergoing surgical procedures, the critical care nurse must understand the potential for electromagnetic interference and monitor postoperatively for appropriate device function.

Critical care nurses are also in a unique position to facilitate do not resuscitate and end-of-life discussions with patients and families. Patients (and families) with CIEDs in situ who are at the end of life (for any cause) are faced with deciding when to deactivate their devices. Critical care nurses should assess patients for endstage disease processes in an effort to support the patients' and families' decisions.[23]

Pharmacotherapeutic Management

Pharmacotherapies used in adjunct to CIED therapy primarily include antiarrhythmics, beta-blockers, and calcium-channel blockers in patients with preserved ejection fractions. Critical care nurses will administer these classes of medications intravenously for acute needs and orally for chronic maintenance.

Nonpharmacotherapeutic Management

Whether it is immediately postoperative or long after CIED placement, all critically ill patients with implanted devices should have infection control measures applied to their care. Critically ill patients requiring invasive lines accessing the bloodstream (eg, central venous catheters, arterial lines, mechanical assist devices) are especially vulnerable for nosocomial microorganisms seeding CIED hardware. Critical care nurses with CIED in situ patients diagnosed with infections should be sure to identify the type of device the patient has and communicate this information to the infectious diseases specialist and/or the attending medical provider.

Other nonpharmacotherapeutic management includes hemodynamic monitoring, surgical site care, and patient and family education.

Patient and family education

There is a saying among nurses who work within hospitals that discharge planning starts at admission. This saying also applies to patients admitted to critical care units for postoperative management of CIED placement. Critical care nurses should anticipate that CIED education began before placement and their role is to build on that knowledge postoperatively until the patient is discharged. **Box 1** is a list of patient education topics that should be discussed with CIED patients.

Patients and families report improved anxiety, depression, quality of life, and other physical outcomes when they receive adequate CIED education.[24] Yildiz and colleagues[24] report events of induced device malfunction can be reduced with a structured education program implemented during early cardiac rehabilitation. Induced device malfunction involves device damage caused by preventable traumatic injury (eg, dislodgement, lead fracture, lead displacement) and electromagnetic radiation.

For the last decade, CIED cybersecurity against hacking has become a concern.[25] The threat of cardiac device hacking can be fatal in some patients. Clinicians must educate patients of the importance of software upgrades as a routine part of care

---

Box 1
Postoperative cardiac implantable electronic device placement patient and family education

- Signs and symptoms of device malfunction
- Signs and symptoms of device infection
- Potential device complications
  - Electromagnetic interference
  - Safe equipment use
- When to go to the emergency department
- Activity of daily living restrictions (particularly device-side extremity use)
- Telemonitoring device use and routine
- Office appointment follow-up schedule
- Palliative care or end-of-life decisions
- Cybersecurity

---

aimed to reduce these vulnerabilities. Other strategies the device manufacturers take against cybersecurity threats should also be discussed with the patient, his or her family, and the cardiology specialist.[26]

SUMMARY

Postoperative CIED placement critical care patients are most often older adults with multiple comorbidities who have special needs. Critical care nurses are in unique position to positively affect patient outcomes when greater knowledge of CIED management is applied to an already vulnerable population of patients. As devices continue to evolve, there is a need for future research in the critical care nurse's role in improving postoperative CIED management.

REFERENCES

1. Hussein AA, Tarakji KG, Martin DO, et al. Cardiac implantable electronic device infections: added complexity and suboptimal outcomes with previously abandoned leads. JACC Clin Electrophysiol 2017;3(1):1–9.

2. Tracy CM, Epstein AE, Darbar D, et al. 2012 ACCF/AHA/HRS focused update of the 2008 guidelines for device-based therapy of cardiac rhythm abnormalities: a report of the American College of Cardiology Foundation/American Heart Association Task Force on practice guidelines. J Am Coll Cardiol 2012;60(14):735–1097.

3. Benjamin EJ, Virani SS, Callaway CC, et al. Heart disease and stroke statistics-2018 update: a report from the American Heart Association. Circulation 2018;1–426. https://doi.org/10.1161/CIR.0000000000000558.

4. Puette JA, Ellison MB. Pacemaker. In: StatPearls [Internet]. Treasure Island (FL): StatPearls Publishing; 2018. Available from: https://www.ncbi.nlm.nih.gov/books/NBK526001/. Accessed October 27, 2018.

5. Reddy VY, Exner DV, Cantillon DJ, et al. Percutaneous implantation of an entirely intracardiac leadless pacemaker. N Engl J Med 2015;373(12):1125–35.

6. Epstein AE, DiMarco JP, Ellenbogen KA, et al. ACC/AHA/HRS 2008 guidelines for device-based therapy of cardiac rhythm abnormalities- a report of the American

College of Cardiology/American Heart Association Task Force on practice guide-lines. J Am Coll Cardiol 2008;51(21):1–62.

7. Medtronic. Micra transcatheter pacing system indications. Medtronic; 2018. Available at: http://www.medtronic.com/us-en/healthcare-professionals/products/cardiac-rhythm/pacemakers/micra-pacing-system/indications-safety-warnings.html. Accessed November 7, 2018.

8. Berg DD, Vaduganathan M, Upadhyay GA, et al. Cardiac implantable electronic devices in patients with left ventricular assist systems. J Am Coll Cardiol 2018; 71(13):1483–94.

9. Bernstein AD, Daubert J-C, Fletcher RD, et al. The revised NASPE/BPEG generic code for antibradycardia, adaptive-rate, and multisite pacing. Pacing Clin Electrophysiol 2002;25(2):260–4.

10. American Heart Association. Implantable cardioverter defibrillator (ICD). American Heart Association; 2016. Available at: http://www.heart.org/en/health-topics/arrhythmia/prevention–treatment-of-arrhythmia/implantable-cardioverter-defibrillator-icd. Accessed November 7, 2018.

11. Kirkfeldt RE, Johansen JB, Nohr EA, et al. Complications after cardiac implant-able electronic device implantations: an analysis of a complete nationwide cohort in Denmark. Eur Heart J 2014;35:1186–94.

12. Udo EO, Zuithoff NP, van Hemel NM, et al. Incidence and predictors of short- and long-term complications in pacemaker therapy: the FOLLOWPACE study. Heart Rhythm 2012;9:728–35.

13. Hussein AA, Baghdy Y, Wazni OM, et al. Microbiology of cardiac implantable electronic device infections. JACC Clin Electrophysiol 2016;2(4):498–505.

14. Dolley YL, Thuny F, Mancini J, et al. Diagnosis of cardiac device-related infective endocarditis after device removal. JACC Cardiovasc Imaging 2010;3(7):673–81.

15. Cerceo E, Deitezweig SB, Sherman BM, et al. Multidrug-resistant gram-negative bacterial infections in the hospital setting: overview, implications for clinical prac-tice, and emerging treatment options. Microb Drug Resist 2016;22(5):412–31.

16. American Heart Association, Devices that may interfere with ICDs and pace-makers. 2016. [Online]. Available at: https://www.heart.org/en/health-topics/arrhythmia/prevention–treatment-of-arrhythmia/devices-that-may-interfere-with-icds-and-pacemakers. Accessed November 6, 2018.

17. Crossley GH, Poole JE, Rozner MA, et al. The Heart rhythm society (HRS)/Amer-ican Society of Anesthesiologists (ASA) expert consensus statement on the peri-operative management of patients with implantable defibrillators, pacemakers and arrhythmia monitors: facilities and patient management this document was developed as joint project with the American Society of Anesthesiologists (ASA), and in collaboration with the American Heart Association (AHA), and the Society of Thoracic Surgeons (STS). Heart Rhythm 2011;8(7):1114–54.

18. Al-Khatib SM, Stevenson WG, Ackerman MJ, et al. 2017 AHA/ACC/HRS guideline for management of patients with ventricular arrhythmias and the prevention of sudden cardiac death: a report of the American College of Cardiology/American Heart Association Task Force on clinical practice guidelines and the hea. J Am Coll Cardiol 2017;72(14):e91–220.

19. Levy WC, Hellkamp AS, Mark DB, et al. Improving the use of primary prevention implantable cardioverter-defibrillator therapy with validate patient-centric risk es-timates. J Am Coll Cardiol 2018;4(8):1089–103.

20. Powell BD, Saxon LA, Boehmer JP, et al. Survival after shock therapy in implant-able cardioverter-defibrillator and cardiac resynchronization therapy-defibrillator

recipients according to rhythm shocked. The ALTITUDE survival by rhythm study. J Am Coll Cardiol 2013;62(18):1674.

21. American Heart Association. Cardiac resynchronization therapy (CRT). American Heart Association; 2018. Available at: https://www.heart.org/en/health-topics/heart-failure/treatment-options-for-heart-failure/cardiac-resynchronization-therapy-crt. Accessed November 8, 2018.

22. Turagam M, Vuddanda V, Velagapudi P, et al. Uninterrupted non-vitamin K antagonist oral anticoagulants versus warfarin in patients undergoing cardiac implantable electronic device implantation: a meta-analysis. J Am Coll Cardiol 2017; 69(11):361.

23. Lambert R, Hayes DL, Annas GJ, et al. HrS expert consensus statement on the management of cardiovascular implantable electronic devices (CIEDs) in patients nearing end of life or requesting withdrawal of therapy. Heart Rhythm 2010;7:1008–26.

24. Yildiz BS, Findikoglu G, Alihanoglu YI, et al. How do patients understand safety for cardiac implantable devices? importance of postintervention education. Rehabil Res Pract 2018;2018:5689353.

25. Baranchuk A, Refaat MM, Patton KK, et al. Cybersecurity for cardiac implantable electronic devices: what should you know? J Am Coll Cardiol 2018;71(11):1284–8.

26. Slotwiner DJ, Deering TF, Fu K, et al. Cybersecurity vulnerabilities of cardiac implantable electronic devices: communication strategies for clinicians - proceedings of the Heart Rhythm Society's Leadership Summit. Heart Rhythm 2018;15:e61–7.

Atrial Fibrillation

Monique Young, ACNP-BC

KEYWORDS

- Atrial fibrillation • Apixaban • Rivaroxaban • Dabigatran

KEY POINTS

- Atrial fibrillation is a growing medical concern that is increasing health care costs and patient unexpected costs.
- The incidence of stroke associated with atrial fibrillation can be decreased with proper education and management.
- There are basic tests such as electrocardiograms, remote telemetry monitoring, and teaching patients how to palpate the pulse to help identify irregularity of pulse.
- Newer anticoagulation medications are now available, including Apixaban, Rivaroxaban, and Dabigatran.
- Nursing plays a vital role in education and prevention.

BACKGROUND

Epidemiology: Prevalence and Significance of Atrial Fibrillation and Anticoagulation

Atrial fibrillation is recognized as the most common arrhythmia and 70% of patients living in the United States with atrial fibrillation are between the ages of 65 to 85 years old. The average age at diagnosis is 75 years old. In 2010, an estimated 5.2 million people were diagnosed with atrial fibrillation. Studies predict that by 2030 an estimated 12.1 million people will be diagnosed with atrial fibrillation. The prevalence of this arrhythmia increases with age, especially in those greater than 50 years of age.[1] For every decade beyond 60 years old, the incidence of atrial fibrillation doubles. The prevalence of atrial fibrillation between men and women is the same, except after age 75, when women have a higher incidence.[1] Women and Medicare patients who are diagnosed with atrial fibrillation also have an increased risk of myocardial infarction and heart failure.[2] The incidence of atrial fibrillation after cardiac surgery is approximately 30%. The lifetime risk of developing atrial fibrillation is 1 in 4.[3] Other comorbidities that increase the incidence of atrial fibrillation are congestive heart failure, hypoxemia, valvular heart disease, and hyperthyroidism.[4] The mnemonic PIRATES spells out the factors predisposing patients to atrial fibrillation (**Box 1**).

No financial or commercial disclosures. No conflicts of interest.
Disclosure: The Author has nothing to disclose.
Louisiana Heart Center, 901 East Gause Boulevard, Slidell, LA 70458, USA
E-mail address: Monique.young@laheart.org

Box 1	
PIRATES	
	Predisposing Factors
P	Pericarditis, pulmonary disease, pulmonary embolism, postoperative
I	Ischemia, infection
R	Rheumatic heart disease (particularly mitral valve disease)
A	Alcohol ("holiday heart), atrial myxoma
T	Thyrotoxicosis, theophylline
E	Enlargement (particularly left atrial enlargement
S	Systemic hypertension, sick sinus syndrome, sleep apnea, and size (obesity)

Atrial fibrillation accounts for one-third of cardiac arrhythmia hospitalizations.[5] A 24-hour ambulatory electrocardiogram study of older patients showed atrial fibrillation in 10% of those who had no prior diagnosis.[6] According to a 2015 study by Ali and associates,[7] the direct medical acute care cost of patients hospitalized with atrial fibrillation is 50% more than those in sinus rhythm. Through years of research, atrial fibrillation has been associated with a 5-fold increase risk of preventable stroke and is a leading cause of death; therefore, atrial fibrillation treatment has become a major health concern. An estimated 15% to 25% of ischemic strokes are associated with atrial fibrillation. Often, stroke is the first presentation and manifestation of atrial fibrillation.[6]

In patients who are diagnosed with atrial fibrillation 25% to 65% of patients are not prescribed anticoagulants.[1] Approximately two-thirds of strokes may be avoided by use of an anticoagulant, which inhibits the formation of blood clots.[7] Deciding to initiate therapy is crucial and the risk of bleeding should be evaluated carefully and assessed by the clinician. Until approximately 2010, warfarin (Coumadin), which inhibits vitamin K (factors II, VII, IX, X, and protein C and S; **Fig. 1**) was the only anticoagulant available. Warfarin has a very narrow therapeutic window and interacts with food, medication, and needs frequent monitoring of the prothrombin time (international normalized ratio [INR]). Warfarin is also associated with increased risk of intracranial hemorrhage (ICH), especially in patients with a higher CHADsVASc score.[8] CHADsVASc is an acronym for a scoring system that evaluates stroke risk and anticoagulation guidance. C is for congestive heart failure (1 point), H is for hypertension (1 point), A is for age greater than 75 (2 points), D is diabetes (1 point), S is for prior stroke, transient ischemic attack, or venous thromboembolism (2 points), V is for vascular disease (peripheral artery disease, myocardial infarction, aortic plaque; 1 point), age 65 to 74 years (1 point), and female sex (1 point). In the last several years, newer agents known as direct oral anticoagulants (DOACs) have been made available. These agents inhibit either factor Xa or thrombin. The newer medications have fewer medication and food interactions and do not require routine laboratory monitoring. The factor Xa inhibitor agents are Apixaban, Rivaroxaban, and edoxaban (see **Fig. 1**). The only oral direct thrombin inhibitor is Dabigatran and is currently the only agent with an antidote approved by the US Food and Drug Administration.[7] Andexanet alfa (Andexxa) is a Xa antidote that is now available in the United States.[8]

When patients are anticoagulated according to standard of care, their risk of death decreased to 19% versus those who were not properly medicated and the 1-year risk of death was 31%.[9] So, why are patients not prescribed anticoagulants given the increased risk of stroke? Reasons why patients are not prescribed an anticoagulant

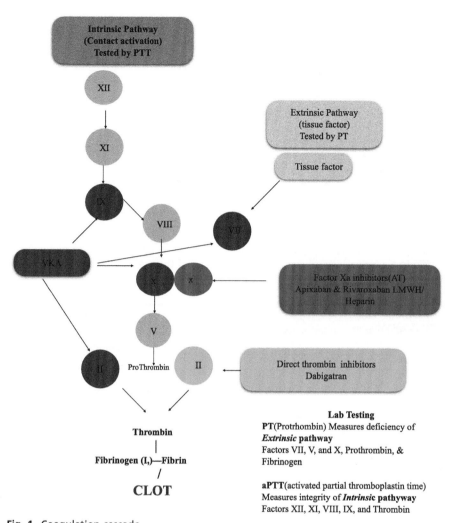

Fig. 1. Coagulation cascade.

is a challenge in treatment; in addition, anticoagulants are associated with 41% of adverse drug events.[9] Warfarin is the second most commonly reported drug in the emergency room for adverse drug events and is on the BEERs list.[8] The BEERs list is a list of medications that carry a higher recommendation to avoid use or limit use in patients greater than 65 year old because they may increase the risk of worsening renal impairment, increase fall risk, and exacerbate ulcers or heart failure. Well-known scoring systems known as CHA_2Ds_2VASc (**Tables 1** and **2**) and HAS-BLED (**Table 3**) are scoring systems that when used give clinicians possible stroke risk and bleeding risk over a 1-year follow-up and assist in initiating and guiding appropriate medical therapy. HAS-BLED scoring has been studied and proven to assist in assessing the risks of stroke and bleeding. The CHA_2Ds_2VASc helps to estimate stroke risk. Studies have shown that, as the CHA_2Ds_2VASc score increases, the risk of ischemic stroke increases proportionately. Persons with a CHA_2Ds_2VASc score of 0 points are considered low risk and aspirin 325 mg/d is considered standard of care rather than other

Table 1 CHA$_2$DS$_2$-VASc risk criteria	
	Points
Congestive heart failure	1
Hypertension	1
Age >75 years	2
Diabetes mellitus	1
Prior stroke/TIA/thromboembolism	2
Peripheral vascular disease/CAD	1
Age 65–74 years	1
Sex (female)	1
Score	10

Abbreviations: CAD, coronary artery disease; TIA, transient ischemic attack.

anticoagulants. However, a score of 0 still calculates an annual risk of stroke (0.8%–3.2%). In 1 study, 10% of patients with a score of 0 were found to have left atrial appendage thrombi on transesophageal echocardiogram.[10]

Table 2 CHA$_2$DS$_2$VASc score	
	Medication Therapy
0	No therapy preferred[a]
1	Aspirin 8–325 mg, or oral anticoagulant[b]
≥2	Oral anticoagulant

[a] If no history of coronary artery disease or <65 years old.
[b] If Warfarin is used and the international normalized ratio should be 2.0 to 3.0 (2.5 is the goal).

Table 3 HAS-BLED	
HAS-BLED	Score
Hypertension that is uncontrolled	1
Abnormal renal/liver function	1 or 2
Stroke	1
Bleeding tendency or predisposition	1
Labile international normalized ratio	1
Age >65 years	1

Drugs (eg, concomitant aspirin,
  or nonsteroidal anti-inflammatory
  drugs) or alcohol
	1

Maximum score	9

Pathophysiology of Coronary Conduction and Pathophysiology of Atrial Fibrillation

Coronary conduction differs from other muscle tissues; the myocardium of the heart encompasses its own system. Specialized cells make up the myocardium and these electrical impulses (cardiac action potential; **Fig. 2**) stimulate electrical impulses to pass from cell to cell stimulating muscle fibers to shorten and relax. The heart is made up of the autonomic system, but neuronal impulses are not necessary to maintain a cardiac cycle. The specialized cells located in nodes are finely tuned and beat in the absence of neuronal stimulation. The sympathetic and parasympathetic nervous systems affect the speed. Cells in each area depolarize at different rates in atrial fibrillation.[11]

The normal path of the heart's conduction system originates in the sinoatrial (SA) node located at the junction of the right atrium and superior vena cava just above the tricuspid valve and beneath the visceral pericardium, making this node very susceptible to injury and/or inflammation (**Fig. 3**). The SA node is also referred to as the pacemaker of the heart and the average action potential of the SA node is 75 beats per minute. During activation of the atrioventricular (AV) node, each myocyte travels through the atria causing depolarization (contraction) of the atria and this is the beginning of systole. The next activation of the cardiac cycle occurs as cardiac cells pass through the AV node located in the right atrial wall above the tricuspid valve. In this area, the cells do not conduct as fast as the SA node, and there is a delay in passing

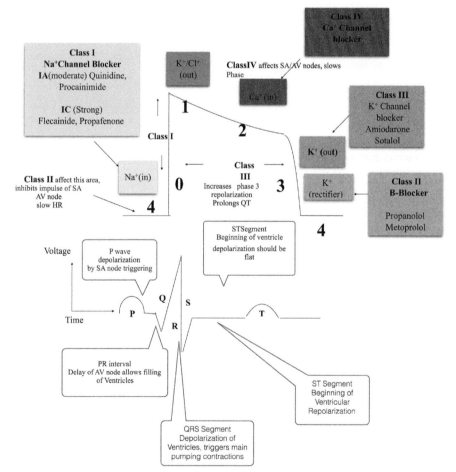

Fig. 2. Drugs affecting the cardiac action potential. Cardiac action potentials (AP) occur only in the sinoatrial (SA) node and atrioventricular (AV) node.

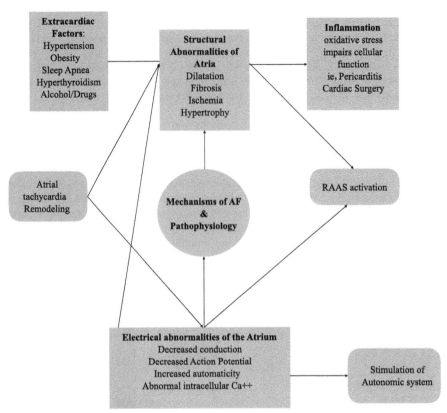

Fig. 3. Factors that increase incidence of AF and RAAS. AF, atrial fibrillation; RAAS, renin–angiotensin–aldosterone system.

of action potential which then proceeds to conduct to the bundle of His and finally through the bundle branches. When cardiac muscles shorten (contract) and relax this is known as systole and diastole. During diastole, the left ventricle is filling (preload) and the atrium muscle is contracting, and during systole, the ventricles are contracting pushing blood to the body (ie, cardiac output).[11]

As stated, atrial fibrillation is characterized by disorganized electrical conduction that originates in 1 or more of the pulmonary veins. There are no discernible P waves, the PR interval is not measurable (wavy baseline), the QRS complex is regularly irregular, the atrial rate is commonly 300 to 400 beats per minute or greater, and the ventricular rate is usually 100 to 160 beats per minute or greater.[4] Given the differing atrial refractory periods of the left atrium to the right atrium, this phenomenon leads to an irregularity of conduction and this leads to a classic fibrillatory conduction in the atrium. The fibrillatory conduction can be seen on an electrocardiogram as disorganized. The ventricular heart rate of atrial fibrillation is variable and the rate is slower than the atria because of a built-in delay.[11]

Atrial fibrillation is common in patients with structural heart disease. Remodeling of the atrium occurs with longer periods of persistent atrial fibrillation, causing shortening of the atrial action potential and refractory period. There is an increased cardiac autonomic tone, which causes dilation of the atria, leading to atrial fibrosis influencing conduction through the atrium, which can trigger atrial fibrillation. Atrial fibrillation increases myocardial demand, decreases filling time, and decreases mean arterial pressure;

therefore, patients with left ventricular dysfunction, left ventricular hypertrophy from uncontrolled hypertension, restrictive cardiomyopathy, or hypertrophic cardiomyopathy decompensate. The loss of AV synchrony impacts ventricular filling times, which is already affected. There is a loss of atrial filling (left ventricular end-diastolic pressure), reducing stroke volume. Although the left ventricular end-diastolic pressure filling is lost, there is an increase of left atrial diastolic pressure, which may lead to pulmonary edema and/or hypotension. Because cardiac output can be affected, coronary blood flow can also be affected, and this is why some patients with atrial fibrillation report chest pain with demand rates and a normal coronary angiogram.[12]

Mortality dramatically increases with patients who develop heart failure from uncontrolled atrial fibrillation. The dyssnychronous rhythm combined with tachycardia predisposes patients to heart failure. Heart disease and atrial fibrillation have been linked to inflammation, which leads to changes in cellular processes. The changes in cellular processes leads to remodeling of the heart's myocardium.[13]

NURSING IMPLICATIONS

Atrial fibrillation is now identified as one of the most costly diseases if not managed correctly. Data suggest that atrial fibrillation is not identified early and is often managed poorly. Managing patients with atrial fibrillation is time consuming and, in today's medical world, time is of the essence and limited. In certain geographic regions, nurse-led clinics have led to improved patient outcomes and decreased mortality and morbidity. Nurse practitioners can educate patients, construct a treatment plan, and protect patients from catastrophic events until mobilization into specialty clinics.[14]

Nursing Intervention and Nursing Communication

The critical care nurse and the nurse practitioner play a significant role in assisting in educating patients and families. Nurses and the advance practitioner knowledgeable about atrial fibrillation may assist in disease management and prevention of complications. Education and knowledge of atrial fibrillation identification and treatment has resulted in a decrease in mismanaged cases of atrial fibrillation which may result in a decrease of mismanaged cases of atrial fibrillation and decreased hospitalizations from atrial fibrillation complications. The nurse is the patient advocate; calling the health care provider with changes in electrocardiogram tracings, calling the health care provider with updated INR results or a change in patient symptoms or clinical stability or instability is crucial. Management of a patient in atrial fibrillation who has other comorbidities, especially with an underlying cardiomyopathy, lung disease, renal disease, cardiovascular disease, and so on.

The disease process can be challenging, but if the nurse/nurse practitioner is knowledgeable, and skillfully trained then early identification, treatment, and management of atrial fibrillation can be simplified. Deescalating medications such as stopping aspirin if it poses no clinically significant adverse outcome is one measure to decrease patient's bleeding risk or teaching avoidance of the use of nonsteroidal anti-inflammatory drugs while using anticoagulants. More aggressive management of hypertension is another measure that increases a patient's bleeding risk; patient education of nonpharmacologic ways to decrease blood pressure would help to decrease the risk associated with increased bleeding.[15]

Nursing Assessment

As stated elsewhere in this article, electrocardiograms are essential in the diagnosis of cardiac arrhythmias; using a systematic approach lessens misdiagnosis, which can lead to a delay in treatment or increased catastrophic events. The correct assessments guide appropriate therapy and avoidance of strokes. Knowing the patient's baseline electrocardiogram is very important. Is this atrial fibrillation new onset or chronic? If it is a new onset atrial fibrillation, then prescribing the appropriate medication to prevent stroke and control rates is important. Also, investigating why the patient may have gone into atrial fibrillation such as sleep apnea, alcohol binge, ischemia, and so on is important. The following questions can help in this investigation. If the diagnosis is known, then is the patient symptomatic? Does the patient feel her or his pulse racing or feel dizzy because of overmedication? Is the patient on anticoagulation, if indicated, and if the patient is not taking an anticoagulant, then why not?

Another assessment and skill needed is palpating the pulse and identifying an irregularity. Palpating the pulse is an easy measure nurses can teach patients. Instruct a normal pulse rate should average 60 to 90 beats per minute and be regular. Early detection is of utmost importance, as well as timing of onset, duration, and any associated symptoms or triggers. Identifying any coexisting disorders, especially underlying cardiac disease and social habits, is important. Screening for alcohol use must be done, because it is not only a risk factor for atrial fibrillation, but also a cause of cardiomyopathy. Common symptoms patients report who have been diagnosed with atrial fibrillation include palpitations, shortness of breath, fatigue, decreased exertional stamina, and chest pressure/pain. Less common symptoms include syncope, but syncope can occur in those diagnosed with sick sinus syndrome and syncope may be the patient's presenting chief complaint. Many occurrences of atrial fibrillation are asymptomatic.[16]

Assess the Patient's Symptoms

The following symptoms may be present:

- Heart palpitations, which may be described as pounding, fluttering, skipping or racing. Some may report "a pain" in their chest.
- Lack of energy, more tired than usual.
- Shortness of breath: patients may be short of breath because their heart is racing or because they are in heart failure, which may change the medication approach and urgency of cardioversion and medication.
- Assessing for a goiter, indicating hyperthyroidism and need for a referral to endocrinology.
- Monitoring the INR. The usual range is 2.0 to 3.0 (optimal is 2.5). The INR is typically monitored frequently until stable and then every 4 to 12 weeks, depending on clinical circumstances.

ROLE OF THE NURSE PRACTITIONER

The management of atrial fibrillation is prevention of stroke. Anticoagulants are a Class I indication in patients with stroke risk of 2 or greater according to CHA_2DS_2-VASc risk tool. An easy way to understand a patient's risk of stroke is to use the CHA_2DS_2-VASc score and double the result. For example, if the sum of the score is 2, then the patient's risk of stroke is 4%.

If the onset of atrial fibrillation is unknown, then rate control medications are used and avoid antiarrhythmic drugs because the possibility of embolic events increases. The patient is then rate controlled with nondihydropyridine calcium channel blockers such as diltiazem (Cardizem) or cardioselective beta-blockers such as metoprolol succinate or esmolol until proper anticoagulation is initiated and expert consult obtained. Beta-blockers decrease the force of the ventricular contraction and increase filling time. Amiodarone is the only antiarrhythmic indicated for patients with a (cardiomyopathy) reduced ejection fraction.[3]

A patient may undergo a transesophageal echocardiogram and when an atrial thrombus is ruled out, then either chemically cardioverted with amiodarone or direct current cardioversion. If the time of onset is known, then to convert the rhythm use amiodarone 1 mg/min for 6 hours and 0.5 mg/min for 18 hours. Another method of converting patients is direct current cardioversion. Anticoagulation is continued for a minimum of 4 weeks or longer after cardioversion. The INR should be maintained at 2 to 3 and, if using the novel anticoagulants, then prescribe according to prescribers insert. The 2014 American Heart Association/American College of Cardiology/Heart Rhythm Society atrial fibrillation guidelines state that ablation is a reasonable first- and second-line therapy for patients diagnosed with symptomatic paroxysmal atrial fibrillation (class I). For those patients with symptomatic persistent atrial fibrillation (class IIa) who have failed antiarrhythmic therapy, ablation is also a second-line therapy.[5] Studies have shown that ablations have decreased atrial fibrillation symptoms but have not been shown to decrease mortality or morbidity.[3]

BLEEDS
Managing Major Bleeds

Dabigatran is the only oral anticoagulant that can be removed by hemodialysis and was the only DOAC with an approved antidote. The cost of the antidote is approximately $5000 and is generally readily available in institutions. Other options to stop major bleeds (this is considered a decrease in the hemoglobin of $\geq$2 g/L and/or transfusion) 5 g of idarucizumab as a fixed-dose intravenous infusion of two 2.5-g aliquots[17] or use of an antifibrinolytic agent, such as tranexamic acid and epsilon aminocaproic acid. Support of hemodynamics. If patient is taking a vitamin K antagonist only 4-factor prothrombin complex concentrates are licensed for rapid vitamin K antagonist reversal and are costly. Prothrombin complex concentrate contain purified vitamin K–dependent clotting factors obtained from pooled human plasma and are free of viral contaminants.[18,19]

Minor Bleeds

Reversal of anticoagulants is not recommended for minor bleeds. Monitor blood counts and signs and symptoms of bleeding: increased heart rate, hypotension, and skin perfusion.[18] If reversal agents are used, then an awareness of the potential for recurrent or worsening of pulmonary embolism, stroke, and deep vein thrombosis needs to be monitored.[8]

Rate Control Versus Rhythm Control

Guidelines are controversial and recommended target heart rate is less than 80 beats per minute. In the RACE II study, lenient rate control of 110 beats per minute versus stricter control of 80 beats per minute was noninferior with respect to cardiovascular mortality and morbidity.[20]

Inpatient and Outpatient Management

Box 2 describes inpatient and outpatient management strategies.

Laboratory tests

If the patient is currently taking Dabigatran, testing the TT, ECT, and ECA may be helpful and contribute to bleeding or surgical risk if emergent (**Fig. 4**). If patient is using

---

Box 2
Inpatient and Outpatient Management Strategies

Strategy	Rationale
Electrocardiogram or rhythm strip	Evaluate for atrial fibrillation, LVH, prior MI[3]
24–48 h Holter monitor	Useful to evaluate patients in the outpatient setting. Correlation of patient's symptoms of palpitations. If rates of atrial fibrillation and if any underlying electrical disorders such as sick sinus syndrome or tachycardia-bradycardia arrhythmia can be identified.[3]
Event recorder	Can be prescribed 7–30 d. Several types: real-time data or one that results are not available till device is brought or mailed back to the monitoring company. Monitors allow immediate data to evaluate medication therapy, response to medication, and atrial fibrillation burden.[3]
Echocardiogram	Used to evaluate the size of the atria and ventricles and detect valvular heart disease[3]
Transesophageal echocardiogram	Much more sensitive and specific test to evaluate left atrial thrombi[3]
Chest radiography	Helpful to assess for pulmonary pathology and assess cardiac borders for enlargement of heart[3]
OSA	Assess patients for possible undiagnosed OSA.[21]
Education	Avoid common triggers: increased stress, excessive alcohol consumption, caffeine intake, use of decongestions due to phenylephrine, use of recreational drugs, dehydration and sleep deprivation[3]

Abbreviations: EAE, ecarin chromagenic assay; ECT, ecarin clotting time; LVH, left ventricular hypertrophy; MI, myocardial infarction; OSA, obstructive sleep apnea.

Apixaban or Rivaroxaban, then an anti–factor Xa assay can be ordered. The International Society on Thrombosis and Hemostasis recommends a DOAC level of greater than 50 ng/mL if surgery is anticipated in a serious bleeder and a level greater than of 30 ng/mL if bleeding risk is high, but less severe.[18]

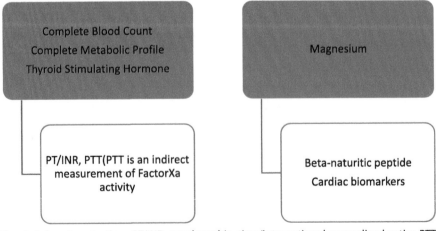

Fig. 4. Laboratory testing. PT/INR, prothrombin time/international normalized ratio; PTT, partial thromboplastin time.

MEDICATIONS: ANTICOAGULATION

When initiating anticoagulation therapy, if warfarin (a vitamin K antagonist) is selected, the baseline INR is needed to assess for underlying coagulopathy. Warfarin at 5 mg/d is a safe starting dose. If inpatient, daily INR testing is recommended; if outpatient start, then monitoring every few days until therapeutic INR and stable warfarin dose is achieved.[18] If using Dabigatran or Rivaroxaban, assess the creatinine clearance. These drugs are dosed according to creatinine clearance. Dabigatran is cleared 85% by the renal system and Rivaroxaban is approximately 33% cleared through the renal system.[3] For patients with a normal creatinine clearance (>50 mL/min), Dabigatran dosing is 150 mg by mouth twice daily and for Rivaroxaban, the dosing is 20 mg/d with a meal. In patients with a creatinine clearance of 30 to 50 mL/min, the dosing for Dabigatran is 75 mg by mouth twice daily. Maximum concentrations of Dabigatran occur 2 to 4 hours after administration.[22] Rivaroxaban prescribed dosing is 15 mg/d and is given with the evening meal. These medications are metabolized in the liver; CYP450 substrate is cleared approximately 27% by the renal system.[3] Maximum concentrations of Rivaroxaban occur 2 to 4 hours after administration.[23]

Dabigatran should be administered with food and a full glass of water to avoid gastric side effects such as dyspepsia or gastritis. Dyspepsia is one of the major complaints of patients, and administering with food and a full glass of water tends to reduce symptoms. Bioavailability and absorption are not affected by administration with food.[22] However, according to the prescriber's insert, the absorption and bioavailability of Rivaroxaban 15 and 20 mg tablets depend on the coadministration of food. Food increases bioavailability from 39% when taken with no food versus 76% with food.[23] Apixaban is dosed based on 3 criteria: age greater than 80 years, weight less than 60 kg, and creatinine of 1.5. Prescribe 2.5 mg by mouth twice daily if patient has 2 out of 3 criteria. Absorption and bioavailability are unaffected by food. This medication is metabolized by the liver; CYP450 substrate.[24] Maximum concentration peaks 3 to 4 hours after ingestion.[3] These medications are not a substitute. Bleeding risks are less when compared with aspirin/clopidogrel or aspirin/warfarin and these medications are not effective in the prevention of stroke.[3]

Holding Anticoagulants

When to hold anticoagulants, if anticoagulants needs to be interrupted, and whether to bridge with low-molecular-weight heparin is not an easy decision. Discrete clinical judgment should be used to guide therapy, including bleeding risks associated with the procedure as well as the patient's thromboembolic risk needs.

According to the ReLy and ROCKET AF trials, there was no increase of stroke or embolism when anticoagulation was interrupted in patients with a CHADs score of 3 or less. However, there was an increased risk of major bleeding complications with bridging for a procedure or surgery. The risk of thromboembolism was less than 0.5%, unlike risk of major bleeding, which was greater than 3%. A patient's bleeding risk with an INR of 1.5 or less the day of the procedure was greater than 2.0% versus a less than 0.5% risk of recurrent venous thromboembolism. For patients who are defined as high risk, guidelines suggest bridging with low-molecular-weight heparin, although there is an associated risk of clinically significant hematoma or bleeding. High risk for atrial fibrillation is defined as a patient whose CHADS score is 4 or greater or who has a prior cerebrovascular accident or transient ischemic attack. The standard of care for patients who had a thrombotic event less than 3 months ago and patients with mechanical heart valves require bridging.

Restarting Anticoagulation

Optimal patient engagement in the decision to restart anticoagulation involves shared decision making with patients and care providers. Determining whether the surgical procedure is a low bleeding risk or high bleeding risk needs to be done. Examples of low bleeding risk procedures include a radial approach angiogram, endoscopy, replacement of pacemaker generator with no lead change, chest tube/thoracentesis, cataract, and carpal tunnel surgery. Examples of high bleeding risk with early administration of anticoagulants are esophageal biopsy, coronary artery bypass grafting, carotid endarterectomy, total hip arthroplasty, and spine surgeries.[18] A full list of procedures can be found in the relevant guidelines. Discussions should include the patient and staff, and encompass the clinical signs of bleeding (eg, monitoring for melena after gastrointestinal bleeding), implications for thrombotic events, and risk of death without anticoagulation.[25] Keep in mind that bleeding risks still are greater than thrombotic risk according to the Rely and ROCKET AF trials. The HAS-BLED scoring system should not be used to stop anticoagulation, but rather to risk stratify a patient. For example, a score of 3 or greater is elevated and these patients may be at increased risk of intracranial bleeding. Educating these patients is prudent.[10]

Initiation of warfarin (a vitamin K antagonist) can be started earlier given that the anticoagulant affect does not begin for 24 to 72 hours. In the BRIDGE trial, the median time to a major bleed was 7.0 days.[18] For the initiation of parenteral anticoagulation, administration recommendation is a minimum of 24 hours for procedures that are deemed la ow bleeding risk and up to 36 to 72 hours for procedures deemed a high risk for bleeding.[18] The administration of parenteral anticoagulation is not necessary if restarting DOACs; treat DOACs like low-molecular-weight heparin.[25]

Oral anticoagulant reinitiation after ICH is a very challenging decision and would involve a multiteam approach, including a neurologist, neurosurgeon, and hematologist. Warfarin-associated ICH are associated with larger ICH and worse mortality. Although DOACs can lead to ICH, the incidence is less than 0.10 to 0.26 cases per 100 person-year.[19] A study trial by Korompoki and colleagues[26] showed resumption of DOACs did not result in recurrent ICH, but a lesser incidence of ischemic stroke.

Rate and Rhythm Medications

Antiarrhythmic medications used to treat atrial fibrillation can be found in several different drug classifications and need careful selection and monitoring. The mechanism of action needs to be understood before prescribing antiarrhythmic medications. Medications that are classified in the classes IA, IC, II, III, and IV are most effective in managing atrial fibrillation (see **Fig. 2**). Ventricular rate control is essential in avoiding increased demand ischemia and heart failure from poorly controlled rate. Now, what does this mean?

Class IA medications include quinidine and procainamide. These medications increase the action potential. These medications increase the QRS and QT intervals. Class IC includes flecainide and propafenone; these medications do not increase or decrease the action potential. These medications increase the QRS interval, slowing the conduction velocity, but have little effect on repolarization. Class II includes beta-blockers (metoprolol, bisprolol, atenolol, etc), which block sympathetic activity, reducing the rate and conduction by decreasing heart rate and increasing the PR interval. Class III includes amiodarone, sotalol, dofetilide, and ibutilide. These medications suppress reentrant rhythms by prolonging the action potential and refractory period and ultimately increase the QT interval. When in the refractory period, cells are too busy to start another action potential, allowing for the filling of ventricles. Class

---

Box 3
Nonpharmacologic therapies

Cardioversion
This can be achieved in 2 ways: by direct electrical current (direct current cardioversion) or antiarrhythmic medication such as amiodarone. Once a patient is cardioverted there is an increased risk of thromboembolism (stunned myocardium) and therefore anticoagulation should be continued for a minimum of 4 weeks.[3]

Surgical management
Given most atrial fibrillation complexes are found near the pulmonary vein, pulmonary vein isolation ablations are done. Maze procedure is another procedure (gold standard).[3]

IV includes nondihydropyridine calcium channel blockers such as diltiazem and verapamil, which impair impulse propagation in nodal and damaged areas and are most effective in reducing rate in conduction of SA and AV nodes. These medications are similar to class II effects and decrease the heart rate and prolong the PR interval.[3]

Other Nonpharmacologic Therapies

Box 3 details other nonpharmacologic therapies.

SUMMARY

Converting to sinus rhythm is more successful when restored early in diagnosis. Risks of atrial fibrillation can be reduced considerably when diagnosed and managed properly. Patients diagnosed with atrial fibrillation can lead and live normal lives exercising. Recurrent hospitalization ultimately increases financial burdens and decreases quality of life.

REFERENCES

1. Badin A, Parr AR, Banga S, et al. Patients' and Physicians' perceptions regarding the benefits of atrial fibrillation ablation. Pacing Clin Electrophysiol 2016;40:362–71.

2. Libby P, Bonow RO, Mann DL, et al. Chapter 75. In: Libby P, Robert RO, Mann DL, et al, editors. Braunwald's heart disease: a textbook of cardiovascular medicine. 8th edition. Philadelphia: Saunders Elsevier; 2010. p. 869–73.

3. Cluculich SP, Kates AM, Defer TM. Cardiology consult subspecialty consult. 3rd edition. St Louis (MO): Wolters Kluwer; 2014.

4. Barkley TW, Myers CM. Practice guidelines for adult gerontological acute care nurse practitioners. 2nd edition. St Louis (MO): Elsevier; 2008.

5. Fuster V, Harrington RA, Narula J, et al. Hurst's the heart. 14th edition. New York: McGraw Hill; 2017.

6. Cavallari I, Patti G. Efficacy and safety of oral anticoagulation in elderly patients with atrial fibrillation. Anatol J Cardiol 2018;19(1):67–71. Available from: Academic Search Complete, Ipswich, MA. Accessed March 7, 2018.

7. Ali AN, Howe J, Abdel-Hafiz A. Cost of acute stroke care for patients with atrial fibrillation compared with those in sinus rhythm. Pharmacoeconomics 2015;33: 511–20.

8. Prescriber's Letter. Anticoagulants, 2018. Available at: https://prescriber. therapeuticresearch.com/Home/PRL.

9. US Department of Health and Human Services, Office of Inspector General. Adverse events in hospitals: national incidence among Medicare beneficiaries. November 2010.

10. Gregory YH, Lip. HAS-BLED Tool – what is the real risk of bleeding in anticoagulation? J Am Coll Cardiol 2012. Available at: http://www.acc.org/latest-in-cardiology/articles/2014/07/18/15/13/has-bled-tool-what-is-the-real-risk-of-bleeding-in-anticoagulation.

11. O'neal WT, Salahuddin T, Broughton ST, et al. Atrial fibrillation and cardiovascular outcomes in the elderly. Pacing Clin Electrophysiol 2016;39:907–13.

12. Rodriguez Y, Althouse A, Adelstein E, et al. Characteristics and outcomes of concurrently diagnosed new rapid atrial fibrillation or flutter and new reduced ejection fraction. Pacing Clin Electrophysiol 2016;39:1394–403.

13. Jaakkola J, Vasankari T, Virtanen R, et al. Reliability of pulse palpation in the Detection of atrial fibrillation in an elderly population. J Prim Health Care 2017;35:293–8.

14. Jacob L. Nurse-led clinics for atrial fibrillation: managing risk factors. Br J Nurs 2017;26:1245–8.

15. Pandya E, Bajorek BV. Assessment of Web-based education resources informing patients about stroke prevention in atrial fibrillation. J Clin Pharm Ther 2016;41:667–76.

16. Scarsoglio S, Guala A, Camporeale C, et al. Impact of atrial fibrillation on the cardiovascular system through a lumped-parameter approach. Med Biol Eng Comput 2014;52:905–20.

17. Pollack CV Jr, Reilly PA, Eikelboom J, et al. Idarucizumab for dabigatran reversal. N Engl J Med 2015;377(17):1691–2.

18. Doherty JU, Gluckman TJ, Hucker WJ, et al. 2017 ACC expert consensus decision pathway for periprocedural management of anticoagulation in patients with nonvalvular atrial fibrillation. J Am Coll Cardiol 2017. https://doi.org/10.1016/j.jacc2016.11.024.

19. Xu Y, Shoamanesh A, AlKherayf F, et al. Oral anticoagulant re-initiation following intracerebral hemorrhage in non-valvular atrial fibrillation: global survey of the practices of neurologists, neurosurgeons and thrombosis experts. PLoS One 2018;13:1–11.

20. McCance K, Huether SE. Pathophysiology: the biological basis for disease in adults children. 8th edition. St Louis (MO): Elsevier; 2018.

21. Zhao E, Chen S, Du Y, et al. Association between sleep apnea hypopnea syndrome and the risk of atrial fibrillation: a meta-analysis of Cohort Study. Biomed Res Int 2018. https://doi.org/10.1155/2018/5215868. Accessed October 22, 2017.

22. Pradaxa. Highlights of prescribing information, 2010. Available at: https://doc.boehringer-ingelheim.com/prescribing%20information/PIs/Pradaxa/Pradaxa.pdf. Accessed October 22, 2017.

23. Xarelto. Highlights of prescribing information, 2011. Available at: http://www.janssenlabels.com/package-insert/product-monograph/prescribinginformation/XARELTO-pi.pdf. Accessed October 22, 2017.

24. Eliquis. Highlights of prescribing information, 2012. Available at: http://packageinserts.bms.com/pi/pi_eliquis.pdf. Accessed October 22, 2017.

25. Hylek EM, Go AS, Chang Y, et al. Effect of intensity of oral anticoagulation on stroke severity and mortality in atrial fibrillation. N Engl J Med 2003;349:1019–26.

26. Korompoki E, Fillippidis FT, Nielson PB, et al. Long-term antithrombotic treatment in intracranial hemorrhage survivors with atrial fibrillation. Neurology 2017;89(7):687–96.

Hospital Discharge Teaching for Patients with Peripheral Vascular Disease

Lucretia M. Wiltz-James, MSN, APRN, FNP-BC*,
James Foley, MSN-HCSM, RN

KEYWORDS

- Peripheral vascular disease • Arteriosclerosis • Atherosclerosis
- Discharge teaching instructions • Life-style modifications

KEY POINTS

- Peripheral disease affects both the arteries and veins.
- Peripheral vascular disease (PVD) is a major problem in the United States, with a high prevalence resulting in both morbidity and mortality.
- PVD is a common disease of the elderly.
- People at greater risk for PVD include smokers, diabetics, those with high blood pressure, and those with elevated cholesterol levels.
- Hospital discharge instructions for patients with PVD include lifestyle modifications; risk reduction therapies, such as antiplatelet, statins, and blood pressure management; and knowing symptoms of disease.

PREVALENCE

Peripheral vascular disease (PVD) is a major problem in the United States, which can lead to loss of limb or even death, PVD has a high prevalence resulting in both morbidity and mortality. Atherosclerosis can appear as early as the first decade of life, with symptoms appearing typically in the fourth or fifth decade of life (**Box 1**).[1] Between 5% and 10% of Americans who are 40 years of age and older are affected with PVD; of those, 40% are smokers.[2] In the age group of 50 years to 59 years, the prevalence of PVD was approximately 3% to 5%; in the age group of 60 years to 69 years, it was 5%; and in those over the age of 80 years, and it was greater than 20% and even greater than 25% in men.[3] In the United States, the rate is similar to those of other developed countries. The mean prevalence rates of PVD in general population for whites, blacks, and

Disclosure Statement: The authors have nothing to disclose.
Louisiana State University Health New Orleans, School of Nursing, 1900 Gravier Street, New Orleans, LA 70112, USA
* Corresponding author.
E-mail address: Ljam14@lsuhsc.edu

Crit Care Nurs Clin N Am 31 (2019) 91–95
https://doi.org/10.1016/j.cnc.2018.11.003
0899-5885/19/© 2018 Published by Elsevier Inc.

Box 1
Risk factors for developing lower extremity peripheral vascular disease

Age

Diabetes

Hyperlipidemia

Diet

Obesity

Smoking

Hypertension

Inflammation

Sedentary lifestyle

Lack of exercise

Asians were 3.5%, 6.7%, and 3.7% respectively.[4] African Americans have a higher prevalence of PAD, even after accounting for other risk factors, and Asian people have a lower prevalence compared with white people. Hispanics may have similar to slightly higher rates of PAD compared with non-Hispanic whites.[4–6] Literature review has suggested that PVD/PAD is a common diagnosis in the aging population.

A vast majority of disorders related to the peripheral vascular system are either atherosclerosis or thrombophlebitis, both affecting the lower extremities more so than the upper extremities or viscera. PVD, also known as arteriosclerosis obliterans, refers to the occlusion or stenosis of arteries, usually occurring in the lower extremities. As the internal lining of the artery thickens from atherosclerotic plaque, the blood vessel becomes increasingly constricted and blood flow diminishes. Atherosclerosis is a chronic inflammatory disease of the arteries that is the most common pathophysiologic process underlying cardiovascular disease (CVD). PVD primary preventions begins by minimizing the risk factors that are controllable, such as eating a healthy diet, maintaining a healthy weight, not smoking, getting regular exercise, and maintaining good control of blood sugar levels to prevent diabetes.[2]

SYMPTOMS

PVD leads to narrowing of blood vessels, which causes a lack of blood supply, most often in the legs and feet. Early in the disease process, blood flow is normal at rest. Symptoms experience depends on what artery is affected and how severely the blood flow is reduced (**Table 1**).[2] As the disease advances, symptoms appear with ambulating for some distance, climbing stairs, or even with mild exercise. The proximal stenosis caused by the atherosclerotic process results in the affected arteries' inability to meet the metabolic blood demands of the distal muscles, subsequently leading to tissue ischemia manifesting in a cramping muscle pain. When a patient rests and ceases exercise, blood supply reaches muscles and pain then subsides. PVD if left untreated can severely debilitate a patient, leading to tissue loss and, in some cases, cause life-threatening infections.[2]

Diagnostic Screening and Testing

PVD is associated with an increased risk of CVD; early diagnosis and management are important. CVD prediction tools, such as the Framingham Risk Score, which is an

Table 1
Symptoms of peripheral vascular disease

Arterial	Venous
• Diminished or absent pulses	• Normal pulses
• Smooth, shiny dry skin, no hair	• Brown patches of discoloration on lower legs
• No edema	• Dependent edema
• Round, regularly shaped painful ulcers on distal foot, toes, or webs of toes	• Irregularly shaped usually painless ulcers on lower legs and ankles
• Dependent rubor	• Dependent cyanosis and pain
• Pallor and pain when legs elevated	• Pain relief when legs elevated
• Intermittent claudication	• No intermittent claudication
• Brittle thick nails	• Normal nails

estimation of 10-year CVD risk of a person, or a questionnaire, such as the Edinburgh Claudication Questionnaire, are good tools to either predict or identify symptoms of PVD.

Diabetic patients are at risk for renal and hepatic impairment post–intravenous contrast mediums. In an effort to prevent complications of contrast medium adverse effects before a procedure, it is best to evaluate the patient's serum creatinine and glomerular filtration rate for elevated results. Complications to avoid contrast medium adverse effects could include hydration through crystalloid infusion and withholding oral forms of diabetic medications for 24 hours.

A more common noninvasive, sensitive screening for PAD is the ankle-brachial index (ABI), a ratio of lower extremity to upper extremity recorded systolic pressures (**Box 2**). ABI is performed by measuring the systolic pressure of the left and right brachial arteries and the left and right posterior tibial and dorsalis pedis arteries pressure. To calculate the ABI, divide the highest pressure in the leg by the highest pressure in the arm. Arterial pressures increase with greater distance from the heart, because of increased arterial impedance as distal arteries taper. Therefore, systolic pressures are normally higher at the ankle than in the brachial arteries, and people without PAD have an ABI of 1.10 to 1.40. An ABI less than 0.90 is approximately 72% sensitive and approximately 99% specific significant for peripheral arterial disease. The ABI may not be accurate in patients with noncompressible arteries.[7,8]

Duplex ultrasound, computerized scan, and nuclear magnetic resonance are other noninvasive diagnostic tools to diagnose PVD. Duplex ultrasound of the lower

Box 2
Ankle-brachial index

- Simple, noninvasive screening
- Normal 0.90
- Less than 0.90 = PAD

$$ABI = \frac{\text{Ankle systolic pressure}}{\text{Brachial systolic pressure}}$$

extremities is cost effective and noninvasive and should be done first to verify stenosis. CT angiography and magnetic resonance angiography is the gold standard for establishing diagnosis but require intravenous contrast. Although screening tools and diagnostic test are important in identifying PVD, for the purpose of this article, diagnostics for PVD are not discussed.

DISCHARGE EDUCATION FOR PATIENTS

For discharge planning to be effective, patient and caregiver education is essential. This can be possible with effective communication between the health care team and the patient as well as the support system. Because hypertension, obesity, sedentary lifestyle, and smoking are some of the predominant risk factors associated with PVD, the registered nurse (RN) and the health care team should focus their attention on these risk factors to help the patient modify lifestyle choices to decrease the risk of PVD occurring. For a behavior change to occur for a patient, the RN needs to focus attention on the patient beliefs regarding current lifestyle and willingness to change.[9] Focusing on a patient's belief system and knowledge base helps the RN understand which areas of education are important and which areas need to emphasized further to help decrease the chances of readmission in the hospital setting.

Once a patient's beliefs and knowledge are understood, effective discharge education can be accomplished with individualized nursing interventions or program development focused on ways to help the patient improve the disease process.[2] The program development should include risk reduction strategies clearly communicated with the patient and/or caregivers included in the process. Two important elements in risk reduction strategies include pharmacologic therapy and behavior modification. In regard to pharmacologic therapy, antiplatelet agents, angiotensin-converting enzyme inhibitors or angiotensinogen receptor blocker, β-blockers, and lipid-lowering agents have shown to reduce the effects of PVD.[10] Because diabetes is also associated as a factor leading to PVD, aggressive monitoring of blood sugars as well as antidiabetic pharmacologic management should be discussed by the health care team regarding compliance, how to afford medication, and administration of medications. Some advantageous behavioral modification strategies should include weight management by tracking weight and physical activity; a healthy diet that consists of eating smaller, more frequent meals; stress reduction teaching; smoking cessation if a patient is a smoker; and decreasing sedentary activities, such as watching television or spending hours on the computer without moving.[2]

These risk reduction interventions can be effective only if a patient and/or caregiver is compliant with the treatment plan. Compliance by patient and/or caregiver can help reduce the risk of PVD complications, such as a loss of a limb, and increase the likelihood for patient survival. This is why the RN and health care team need to encourage patient education upon admission and continue to formulate an individualized treatment plan for the patient. Compliance needs to continue with the health care team throughout the treatment process, including follow-up visits; laboratory tests, such as hemoglobin A_{1c} and fasting glucose levels; and continued patient/caregiver education when necessary.

SUMMARY

Early recognition of signs and symptoms of PVD is vital to an individual's well-being and longer course of life. With effective communication and education by the health care team, an individual can live a long and productive life. By minimizing risk factors, such as smoking, eating a fatty diet, and monitoring hemoglobin A_{1c} with a target goal of less than 7%, this can be attainable. Education is a vital component to prevention in the less privileged areas of America. The extensive literature review strongly suggests prevention is essential, especially understanding patients' education and economic backgrounds. This can help health care providers determine type of medication administration, food options, and exercise regimen that individuals can afford. RNs must take an active role in discharge planning for individual patients in the inpatient as well as outpatient setting to help produce effective results for their patients. The health care team should also monitor self-care adherence to determine the best results for patients with PVD.

REFERENCES

1. Tuzcu EM, Kapadia SR, Tutar E, et al. High prevalence of coronary atherosclerosis in asymptomatic teenagers and young adults evidence from intravascular ultrasound. Circulation 2001;103:270502710.
2. Lopes-Costa E, Amato-Vealey E. Identifying beliefs about smoking in patients with peripheral vascular disease. J Vasc Nurs 2016;34(4):137–43.
3. Peripheral arterial disease (PAD) fact sheet. Center for disease control and prevention. Available at: https://www.cdc.gov/dhdsp/data_statistics/fact_sheets/fs_pad.htm. Accessed July 2018.
4. Vitalis A, Lip GY, Kay M, et al. Ethnic differences in the prevalence of peripheral vascular disease: a systematic review and meta-analysis. Expert Rev Cardiovasc Ther 2017;15(4):327–38.
5. Roger VL, Go AS, Lloyd-Jones DM, et al. Heart disease and stroke statistics 2011 update: a report from the American Heart Association. Circulation 2011;123: e18–209.
6. West JA. Cost effective strategies for the management of vascular disease. Vasc Med 1997;2:25–9.
7. McDermott MM, Criqui MH. Ankle-Brachial Index and screening and improving peripheral artery disease and detection and outcomes. JAMA 2018;320(2):143–5.
8. Lijmer JG, Hunink MG, van den Dungen JJ, et al. ROC analysis of noninvasive tests for peripheral arterial disease. Ultrasound Med Biol 1996;22(4):391–8.
9. Patel PV, Gilski D, Morrison J. Improving outcomes in high-risk populations using REACH®. Crit Pathw Cardiol 2009;8(3):112–8.
10. Gerhard-Herman MD, Gornik HL, Barrett C, et al. 2016 American Heart Association/American College of Cardiology Guideline on the management of patients with lower extremity peripheral disease: A report of the AHA/ACC task force on clinical practice guidelines. J Am Coll Cardiol 2017;69(11).

Acute and Chronic Hypertension

What Clinicians Need to Know for Diagnosis and Management

Sherry L. Rivera, DNP, ANP-C[a],*, Jennifer Martin, DNP, CRNA[b],
Jessica Landry, DNP, FNP-BC[c]

KEYWORDS

- Hypertension • Hypertension management • Hypertension detection
- Resistant hypertension management • Emergency management of hypertension
- Hypertension and comorbidities • White coat hypertension
- Pseudoresistant hypertension

KEY POINTS

- Hypertension is a prevalent, treatable cause of cardiovascular disease.
- Improving cardiovascular outcomes is the primary goal of hypertension management and treatment.
- Ten percent of cases of hypertension have secondary causes.
- Accuracy of blood pressure measurement is essential for appropriate diagnosis, management, and treatment of hypertension.
- Hypertensive emergency is associated with acute end organ damage and requires immediate intervention.

INTRODUCTION

Hypertension is the most common primary diagnosis in the United States and is a treatable cause of cardiovascular disease (CVD) morbidity and mortality. According to the American Heart Association (AHA) (2018), 45% of adults in the United States currently have hypertension.[1] Over the past decade, health care costs and the number of deaths related to hypertension have continued to climb.[1] Current estimates

Disclosure Statement: The authors have nothing to disclose.
[a] Nurse Practitioner Program, LSU Health New Orleans School of Nursing, 1900 Gravier Street, New Orleans, LA 70112, USA; [b] Nurse Anesthesia Program, LSU Health New Orleans School of Nursing, 1900 Gravier Street, New Orleans, LA 70112, USA; [c] PCFNP Concentration, LSU Health New Orleans School of Nursing, 1900 Gravier Street, New Orleans, LA 70112, USA
* Corresponding author.
E-mail address: srive4@lsuhsc.edu

Crit Care Nurs Clin N Am 31 (2019) 97–108
https://doi.org/10.1016/j.cnc.2018.11.008
0899-5885/19/© 2018 Elsevier Inc. All rights reserved.

ccnursing.theclinics.com

anticipate the cost of hypertension will reach $221 billion by the year 2035.[1] Although the risk of developing primary hypertension increases with age due to physiologic alterations of one's cardiovascular (CV) structure and functionality, hypertension does occur in pediatric patients as well. Worldwide and in the United States, untreated or uncontrolled hypertension heightens CV risk leading to the onset of vascular and renal damage. Hypertension is an independent risk factor for multiple sequelae of disease states, including myocardial infarction, chronic kidney disease (CKD), ischemic and hemorrhagic stroke, heart failure, and premature death. Meta-analysis evidence indicates that by lowering blood pressure (BP) by as little as 1 to 2 mm Hg that CV-related morbidity and mortality are significantly reduced.[2] Widespread control of hypertension continues to be an elusive challenge despite available evidence and can be a source of frustration for patients and providers. A collaborative effort between patient and clinician using a balance of pharmacologic and nonpharmacologic interventions is essential to effectively manage and treat hypertension to avoid target organ damage and improve health outcomes.

PRIMARY HYPERTENSION
Pathophysiology

The predisposition to idiopathic, or essential hypertension, is polygenic in origin. Full expression of the disease process may be found when combined with behavioral factors, including obesity, decreased physical activity levels, increased stress levels, alcohol consumption, high dietary sodium, or low dietary potassium, calcium, and magnesium. Essentially, hypertension accounts for more than 95% of cases and appears to be caused by a multifaceted interaction between genetic predisposition and the behavioral factors listed previously. This complex interaction seems to affect levels of sodium and catecholamines, the renin-angiotensin system, insulin, and cell membrane function, which all lead to an elevation of the BP.[3]

More common detectible causes of hypertension include the following:

- Chronic renal disease (2%–5%)
- Renovascular disease (0.2%–0.7%)
- Cushing syndrome (0.1%–0.6%)
- Pheochromocytoma (0.04%–0.1%)
- Primary hyperaldosteronism (0.01%–0.30%).[4]

Diagnosis

Because of the high prevalence of hypertension, measurement of BP should be considered at each health care visit. According to Whelton and colleagues,[5] BP measurements are based on an average of 2 or more appropriate measurements obtained on 2 or more independent occurrences (**Table 1** provides parameters defining hypertension). The diagnosis of hypertension is confirmed by a qualified clinician only after BP measurements are obtained using proper technique. Proper technique includes the following:

1. Instructions of abstinence from nicotine and caffeine for at least 30 minutes before the measurement of the BP
2. Use of a mercury sphygmomanometer or a recently calibrated aneroid device
3. Bladder of the BP cuff encircling 80% of the upper arm
4. Measurement taken after at least 5 minutes of rest with the patient sitting, back supported, and arm bared and supported at heart level
5. Two separate readings timed 2 minutes apart are averaged[5]

Table 1			
Diagnostic measurement of blood pressure			
BP Category	**SBP**		**DBP**
Normal	<120 mm Hg	and	<80 mm Hg
Elevated	120–129 mm Hg	and	<80 mm Hg
Hypertension	—		—
Stage 1	130–139 mm Hg	or	80–89 mm Hg
Stage 2	≥140 mm Hg	—	≥90 mm Hg

Individuals with SBP and DBP in 2 categories should be designated to the higher BP category.
From Whelton PK, Carey RM, Aronow WS, et al. 2017 ACC/AHA/AAPA/ABC/ACPM/AGS/APhA/ ASH/ASPC/NMA/PCNA guideline for the prevention, detection, evaluation, and management of high blood pressure in adults: a report of the American College of Cardiology/American Heart Association Task Force on Clinical practice guidelines. J Am Coll Cardiol 2018;71:2209; with permission.

Patient Evaluation

Once the presence of hypertension is confirmed per the diagnostic criteria, the clinician must perform a comprehensive history and physical examination and recommended diagnostic testing, such as urinalysis; complete blood count; lipid profile; serum creatinine with estimated glomerular filtration rate; serum potassium, sodium, and calcium; fasting glucose; and electrocardiogram.[6] The purpose of this evaluation is to identify other CV risk factors, end organ damage, and secondary forms of hypertension (**Table 2**). Secondary forms of hypertension can be identified in approximately 10% of adult patients diagnosed with hypertension. Secondary hypertension should be considered by the clinician when examining younger patients (<30 years of age) with elevated BP measurements.[4] End organ damage is discussed in greater detail in the Hypertensive Emergencies section.

Table 2		
Purpose of evaluation		
Other CV Risk Factors	**End Organ Damage**	**Secondary Forms of Hypertension**
• Smoking • Hyperlipidemia • Diabetes mellitus • Age >60 y • Male • Family history of CVD in a female relative before age 65 y or a male relative before 55 y	• Left ventricular hypertrophy • Angina • Previous myocardial infarction Previous angioplasty or coronary revascularization • Heart failure • Stroke or transient ischemic attack • Nephropathy • Peripheral arterial disease • Retinopathy	• Renal parenchymal disease • Renovascular disease • Primary aldosteronism • OSA • Drug or alcohol induced • Pheochromocytoma/ paraganglioma • Cushing syndrome • Hypothyroidism/ hyperthyroidism • Aortic coarctation (undiagnosed or repaired) • Primary hyperparathyroidism • Congenital adrenal hyperplasia • Mineralocorticoid excess syndromes • Acromegaly

Data from Refs.[4,21,22]

Management

The first step of hypertension management should include an assessment of risk. Information gathered while conducting a comprehensive history can facilitate the identification of modifiable and nonmodifiable risk factors to determine an individual patient's level of risk and the most appropriate plan for treatment. A family history of hypertension can reveal a potential genetic predisposition for developing hypertension. The social history can provide valuable information about smoking, alcohol intake, and the use of illicit drugs. A review of medications can be helpful to identify prescription or over-the-counter medications such as nonsteroidal anti-inflammatory medications that contribute to an elevated BP. Additional factors that can be revealed in a comprehensive history and physical include cultural lifestyle, obesity, level of physical activity, and diet habits. Lifestyle modification, such as smoking cessation, weight loss, exercise, and a low-fat, low-sodium diet, should always be recommended as the first line of treatment and in addition to pharmacologic treatment.

Clinicians have several options when treating a patient with elevated BP measurements and a diagnosis of hypertension has been made. According to the 2017 AHA Clinical Practice Guideline, evidence-based recommendations for practice include the following: (1) "Use of BP-lowering medications is recommended for secondary prevention of recurrent CVD events in patients with clinical CVD and an average SBP (systolic BP) of 130 mm Hg or higher or an average DBP (diastolic BP) of 80 mm Hg or higher, and for primary prevention in adults with an estimated 10-year atherosclerotic cardiovascular disease (ASCVD) risk of 10% or higher and an average SBP 130 mm Hg or higher or an average DBP 80 mm Hg or higher; and (2) use of BP-lowering medication is recommended for primary prevention of CVD in adults with no history of CVD and with an estimated 10-year ASCVD risk less than 10% and an SBP of 140 mm Hg or higher or a DBP of 90 mm Hg or higher."[5]

Clinicians have several classes of antihypertensive agents available to treat their patients with elevated BP measurements (**Table 3**). Pharmacologic agents that have been proven to reduce clinical events should be used preferentially. Although many patients will begin their treatment regimen on a single agent, some will require 2 or more drugs from diverse pharmacologic classes in order to reach their BP goals.[7] The clinician must have vast knowledge of the pharmacologic mechanisms of action of each agent to provide their patient with the best treatment options available. Therefore, drug regimens with balancing activity can result in the synergistic effect resulting in improved patient outcomes.[8]

PSEUDORESISTANT HYPERTENSION

Pseudoresistant hypertension is a term used to describe hypertension that appears to be resistant to treatment but is in reality related to factors that are modifiable. Medication adherence, inaccurate BP measurement technique, poor dietary habits, smoking, alcohol abuse, obesity, white coat hypertension, caffeine, or the use of other stimulants are common causes of pseudoresistance. Insufficient use of antihypertensive medication and medication adherence are the most common causes of pseudoresistance.[9] Approximately 50% of patients with what appears to be resistant hypertension do not take their antihypertensive medications.[10] Forty percent of patients newly diagnosed with hypertension will discontinue the use of antihypertensive medications within 1 year of diagnosis.[11] Poor adherence with antihypertensive medication has been linked to poorer health outcomes and increases the risk of death to 80%.[12] Multiple patient-, provider-, and system-related factors have been identified

Table 3		
Pharmacologic and nonpharmacologic treatments for hypertension		
Pharmacologic		**Nonpharmacologic**
Primary agents	Secondary agents	• Weight loss
• Thiazide or thiazide type Diuretics	• Diuretics: loop	• Heart healthy diet
	• Diuretics: potassium sparing	• Sodium reduction
	• Diuretics: aldosterone antagonists	• Potassium supplementation
• Angiotensin ACE inhibitors	• Beta-blockers: cardioselective	• Increased physical activity
• ARBs	• Beta-blockers: cardioselective and vasodilatory	• Alcohol reduction or abstinence
• CCB: dihydropyridines	• Beta-blockers: non-cardioselective	
• CCB: non-dihydropyridines	• Beta-blockers: intrinsic sympathomimetic activity	
	• Beta-blockers: combined alpha- and beta-receptor	
	• Direct renin inhibitor	
	• Alpha-1 blockers	
	• Central alpha2-agonist and other centrally acting drugs	
	• Direct vasodilators	

that influence adherence with antihypertensive medications. Complex dosing regimens, lack of consistency taking prescribed medications, cost of medications, and negative side effects, such as dizziness, fatigue, and impotence, are commonly cited issues related to medication adherence.[11] Provider continuity of care, feeling connected to a pharmacist, and affordability of medication are the strongest predictors of medication adherence.[13] Communication and collaboration between patient and provider are key aspects of improving medication adherence and management of hypertension. Reducing pill burden and management of side effects related to antihypertensive medications could improve adherence. A thorough review of medications encompassing prescription medications, dietary supplements, and use of over-the-counter medications should also be evaluated when determining the cause of difficult to control hypertension. Commonly prescribed medications, such as decongestants, ephedra, nonsteroidal anti-inflammatory medications, corticosteroids, tricyclic antidepressants, and oral contraceptives, can also contribute to worsening or difficult to control hypertension.

White Coat Hypertension

White coat hypertension should be considered when BP readings are higher in the office than usual readings obtained at home. The prevalence of white coat hypertension ranges from 13% to 35% with non-smoking older women affected more often.[5] Patients with white coat hypertension are at risk for overtreatment of hypertension. Episodes of hypotension and complaints of persistent fatigue should prompt further evaluation for hypertension related to white coat effect.[11] Monitoring BP at home or the use of ambulatory BP monitoring can be useful to rule out white coat hypertension and is a more reliable indication of risk related to CVD than BP readings obtained in the office.[5]

Inaccuracy of Measurement

The accuracy of BP measurement is essential for appropriate diagnosis, management, and treatment of hypertension. Current guidelines by the AHA (2018) for BP measurement are not routinely used in practice.[5] Electronic devices used for determining treatment should be validated for every patient according to the current guidelines by the AHA (2018). Errors in measurement can still occur despite using a validated machine and should be considered when determining source of difficult to control hypertension. Inappropriate cuff size is the most common source of BP error.[5] Arm circumference should be measured annually to ensure appropriate cuff size is used.[5] Routine monitoring of BP should be encouraged and is useful for confirmation and to evaluate effectiveness of treatment. Patients should be educated regarding the appropriate way to monitor BP according to the AHA guidelines (2018).

RESISTANT HYPERTENSION

Hypertension is considered resistant when control is not achieved despite the use of 3 or more complementary antihypertensives with one of which being a diuretic or requiring 4 or more medications to achieve control.[5] Resistant hypertension affects approximately 13% of adults and is likely underestimated according to the recently released clinical practice guidelines by the American College of Cardiology (ACC) and AHA Task Force.[5] Risk factors associated with a higher risk for development of resistant hypertension include obesity, advanced age, diabetes, CKD, and black race.[5] Secondary causes of hypertension should be considered in the presence of severe hypertension, early or sudden onset of hypertension, change in BP from well controlled to elevated, presence of target organ damage disproportionate to duration of hypertension, and resistance after modifiable factors have been addressed.[5] Secondary hypertension accounts for a small percentage of cases of resistant hypertension. Treatment of the underlying cause can result in improvement of hypertension. Primary hyperaldosteronism, renovascular disease, obstructive sleep apnea (OSA), sleep patterns, CKD, and obesity are a few of the most common secondary causes of resistant hypertension.

Primary Hyperaldosteronism

Primary hyperaldosteronism is considered the most common secondary cause of resistant hypertension and affects approximately 20% of patients with resistant hypertension.[5] Individuals with primary hyperaldosteronism are at a higher risk for developing CV and kidney disease.[5] Primary hyperaldosteronism is characterized by hypertension and may be with or without hypokalemia present. A family history of hypertension or cerebral vascular accident at a young age, adrenal adenomas, bilateral adrenal hyperplasia, or slightly elevated serum sodium level are also additional factors that should prompt further workup for this diagnosis.[14,15] Computed tomography (CT) imaging of the adrenal glands can be used to determine if adrenal abnormalities are present.

Primary hyperaldosteronism should be suspected based on an elevated serum aldosterone/renin ratio result of greater than 20 ng/dL with an elevated serum aldosterone level of at least 10 ng/dL. Diagnosis is confirmed based on an aldosterone suppression test.[14,15] Positive results should be referred to endocrinology.[5] Treatment includes the use of mineralocorticoid receptor antagonists, such as spironolactone or unilateral adrenalectomy as indicated.

Renal Artery Stenosis

Renal artery stenosis (RAS) is a narrowing of the renal artery and results in a reduction in renal blood flow.[5] The most common cause of RAS is atherosclerosis. Traumatic, neoplastic, or embolic occlusion can cause unilateral RAS. Thrombosis, vasculitis, and vascular occlusion can cause RAS bilaterally. A reduction in renal blood flow results in activation of the renin-angiotensin-aldosterone system (RAAS) and can contribute to worsening or resistant hypertension over time. Sudden onset of hypertension, malignant hypertension, and pulmonary edema should raise suspicion for the possibility of RAS. The effects of the reduced blood flow may not be evident until at least 70% of the lumen is occluded.[15] Clinical manifestations may include a progressive decline in renal function, an increase in serum creatinine, or acute kidney injury after initiating treatment with an angiotensin converting enzyme inhibitor (ACE inhibitor), asymmetrical kidney size greater than 1.5 cm, and renal artery bruit.

The goals of treatment are to improve hypertension control and to improve CV and renal-related outcomes. Reducing the effect of the RAAS and retention of sodium and water should be the focus of managing hypertension. The combination of beta-blockers and diuretics can blunt the effects of renin. Caution should be used when using ACE inhibitors or angiotensin receptor blockers (ARBs) in the presence of RAS because it may cause a decline in renal function or result in acute kidney injury. A basic metabolic panel should be obtained within 1 week of initiating therapy with an ACE inhibitor or ARB to evaluate for hyperkalemia or further decline in renal function. Calcium channel blockers (CCBs) can be used as alternative therapy when ACE inhibitors or ARBs are contraindicated or not tolerated. Additional treatment should include management of dyslipidemia and diabetes, smoking cessation, and antiplatelets. Revascularization or angioplasty may be used depending on cause and individual patient risk factors.

Sleep Disturbance

Duration of sleep and disturbance in sleep patterns can contribute to higher CV risk and resistant hypertension. Studies have demonstrated that sleeping 5 hours or less has been linked to higher rates of hypertension and all-cause mortality.[16] Lack of sleep or disturbance of sleep blunts the nocturnal dip in BP contributing to the development of hypertension.[15] Adequate sleep and treatment of underlying sleep disturbances have the potential to reduce hypertension and CV risk.

OSA causes disturbance in sleep and is a common finding in individuals with resistant hypertension. OSA affects men more frequently than women. Obesity, aging, history of cardiopulmonary disease or cerebral vascular accident, chronic use of opioids, and neuromuscular disease are additional risk factors.[16] OSA is characterized by collapse of the upper airways resulting in intermittent episodes of apnea, hypoxemia, and hypercapnia. Serum aldosterone levels are directly associated with severity of OSA.[15] A nocturnal shift in fluid due to chronic volume overload is thought to be a contributing factor for the collapse of the upper airways.[15] Sympathetic stimulation, retention of sodium and water, impaired vasodilation, and a chronic underlying inflammatory response contribute to hypertension and heightened CV risk in response to hypoxemia and hypercapnia.[10,15]

A history of snoring, excessive daytime sleepiness, difficulty sleeping, nocturnal gasping, insomnia, and witnessed apneic episodes are common symptoms of OSA.[16] Individuals suspected of having OSA should be referred for a sleep evaluation. Diagnosis is based on polysomnography (PSG) testing. The presence of 5 or more apneic events per hour with reported symptoms or 15 or more apneic events per hour without reported symptoms yields positive results. Treatment is dependent on PSG findings. Weight loss and treatment of OSA with the use of continuous positive airway pressure can improve BP control, reduce aldosterone levels, and improve CV outcomes.[10]

Obesity

The first line of treatment of obesity includes weight loss, diet, and exercise. According to Whelton and colleagues,[5] approximately 40% of all cases of hypertension are related to obesity. A 10% weight gain can increase SBP by almost 7 mm Hg. Weight loss can reduce BP and improve effectiveness of antihypertensive medications.[15] When determining a plan of treatment for resistant hypertension, the metabolic effects of obesity (**Table 4**) and the adverse effect of antihypertensive medications should be considered. Beta-blockers can contribute to weight gain and worsen insulin resistance. Thiazide diuretics should be used in low doses because of their negative impact on insulin resistance. ACE inhibitors and ARBs have a positive effect on insulin resistance. CCBs are also an option because of their metabolically neutral profile.[15]

Chronic Kidney Disease

Resistant hypertension is 3 times more prevalent in the CKD population (~25%) than the population with essential hypertension (~8%) presenting a multifaceted challenge.[17] Uncontrolled hypertension is a primary risk factor for the development of CKD and can contribute to a more rapid progression of kidney disease. By the time renal function has declined to stage 5 CKD, approximately 65% to 95% of the CKD population has developed hypertension.[17] Individuals with CKD are at a higher risk for poor CV outcomes than the general population, making control of hypertension a priority. The presence of microalbuminuria further amplifies CV risk. The primary goal of treatment is to slow the progression of CKD and to reduce poor outcomes related to CVD.

The management of hypertension becomes more challenging as kidney disease progresses. Sustained stimulation of the sympathetic nervous system and RAAS, increased arterial stiffness, vasoconstriction resulting in glomerular hyperfiltration, sodium sensitivity, and impaired sodium and water excretion that worsens as renal function declines contribute to increased intravascular volume and the development of hypertension in CKD. Treatment should focus on suppression of the sustained effects of the RAAS and reduction of fluid volume. Sodium restriction is paramount when treating resistant hypertension in the presence of CKD. ACE inhibitors or ARBs, CCBs, diuretics, and sodium restriction of less than 2 g of sodium per day can effectively reduce BP. The combination of ACE inhibitors and sodium restriction can also reduce albuminuria.[17] Hypotension related to aggressive BP management can cause ischemic changes in the kidney resulting in a more rapid progression of kidney disease.

Pheochromocytoma

Pheochromocytoma is a rare cause of secondary hypertension characterized by excess catecholamines and renin levels. Clinical symptoms prompting consideration

Table 4 Metabolic effects of obesity	
Chronic inflammatory condition	Activation of renin angiotensin aldosterone system
Remodeling of vasculature	Fat deposits in CV system
Decreased ability to vasodilate	Microvascular dysfunction
Increased stimulation of sympathetic nervous system	Development of insulin resistance
Decreased excretion of sodium	

of screening for pheochromocytoma include headaches, tremors, palpitations, diaphoresis, anxiety, hyperglycemia, weight loss, cardiac arrhythmias, and new onset of hypertension that is difficult to control.[15,18] Diagnostic workup includes serum catecholamine levels, 24-hour urine for metanephrine and catecholamine levels, CT, or MRI. Serum catecholamine levels greater than 2000 pg/mL are considered elevated.[18] Surgical resection is the treatment of choice. Treatment with alpha-adrenergic receptor blockers such as phenoxybenzamine is used to manage symptoms and hypertension while surgery is pending.[18] The use of beta-adrenergic blockers can be considered for cardiac symptoms if alpha-adrenergic receptor blockers are ineffective in reduction of symptoms.[18]

HYPERTENSIVE EMERGENCIES

A hypertensive emergency is diagnosed when the BP is greater than 180/120 mm Hg and is associated with evidence of new or worsening end organ damage.[5] Hypertensive urgencies are defined as elevated BP but without evidence of new or worsening end organ damage.[5,19,20] Determining the underlying cause of hypertension urgency is an important distinguishing factor for treatment.[5] Patients with hypertensive urgencies should not be treated with intravenous antihypertensives nor referred to the emergency department.[5]

In the hypertensive emergency, there is a loss of autoregulation of blood flow, and arterioles vasoconstrict to counter the high-pressure gradients.[19] These high pressures easily overcome and damage the small arterioles, specifically causing endothelial injury, which increases permeability of the vessel, activates the body's coagulation cascade, and causes an inflammatory response to ensue.[19] When the renin-angiotensin system is activated, further vasoconstriction is possible and more inflammation within the vessel occurs. End organ damage begins with end organ ischemia, which worsens the inflammatory response.[19] Organs most affected by hypertensive emergencies include the brain, heart, kidneys, retina, and uterus (placenta) in pregnancy.[19]

Cause and Diagnosis

The causes of hypertensive emergencies can be many, including essential hypertension, renal disease, prescribed medications, illegal substances, pain, and pregnancy complications.[19] Other causes could be endocrine in nature, such as a pheochromocytoma, Cushing syndrome, or renin-secreting tumors.[19] Central nervous system disorders, such as head trauma, spinal cord injuries, or brain tumors, can also affect the body's ability to regulate BP.[19] The clinician should immediately assess for signs of end organ damage. The patient should be asked about associated symptoms, such as chest pain, shortness of breath, dizziness, focal weakness or changes in sensory or motor abilities, alterations in mental status, and headaches.[19] The physical examination should be comprehensive and include a neurologic examination to assess for signs of stroke, fundoscopic examinations to assess for papilledema or retinal hemorrhages, and a complete CV assessment. The patient should be examined for jugular venous distention, adventitious breath sounds such as rales, heart murmurs, and peripheral pulses should be symmetric and palpable.[19]

To completely assess for end organ damage, a series of diagnostic studies should be ordered and closely evaluated for changes from previous studies. The complete blood count should be examined for anemia and/or thrombocytopenia.[19] A complete metabolic profile should be examined for elevated blood urea nitrogen/creatinine, elevated liver enzymes, and abnormal electrolyte levels. Consider using a troponin

Table 5
Intravenous antihypertensive drugs for treatment of hypertensive emergencies

Drug and Class	Usual Dose	Comments
Nicardipine CCB: dihydropyridine	Initial 5 mg/h, increasing every 5 min by 2.5 mg/h to maximum of 15 mg/h	Do not use in advanced aortic stenosis. No dose adjustments required in the elderly
Sodium nitroprusside Vasodilator: nitric oxide dependent	Initial 0.3–0.5 μg/kg/min; increase in increments of 0.5 μg/kg/min to achieve BP target. Maximum dose is 10 μg/kg/min. Duration should be as short as possible. Infusion rates ≥4–10 μg/kg/min or duration >30 min. Thiosulfate can be coadministered to prevent cyanide toxicity	Intra-arterial BP monitoring is recommended. Lower doses for elderly. Cyanide toxicity is possible with prolonged use
Nitroglycerin Vasodilator: nitric oxide dependent	Initial 5 μg/min; increase in increments of 5 μg/min every 3–5 min to a maximum of 20 μg/min	Use only in patients with acute coronary syndrome and/or acute pulmonary edema. Avoid in volume-depleted patients
Hydralazine Vasodilator: direct acting	Initial 10 mg via slow intravenous infusion (maximum initial dose 20 mg); repeat every 4–6 h as needed	BP begins to decrease within 10–30 min, and the decrease lasts 2–4 h. Unpredictability of response and prolonged duration of action do not make hydralazine a desirable first-line agent
Esmolol Adrenergic blockers/beta selective	Loading dose 500–1000 μg/kg/min over 1 min followed by a 50 μg/kg/min infusion. For additional dosing, the bolus is repeated and the infusion increased in 50 μg/kg/min increments as needed to a maximum of 200 μg/kg/min	Contraindicated in patients with concurrent beta-blocker therapy. Monitor for bradycardia. May worsen heart failure
Enalaprilat ACE inhibitor	Initial 1.25 mg over a 5-min period. Doses can be increased up to 5 mg every 6 h as needed	Contraindicated in pregnancy. Do not use in acute myocardial infarction. Slow onset of action (15 min) and unpredictable responses. Useful in hypertensive emergencies associated with high-plasma renin activity

From Whelton PK, Carey RM, Aronow WS, et al. 2017 ACC/AHA/AAPA/ABC/ACPM/AGS/APhA/ASH/ASPC/NMA/PCNA guideline for the prevention, detection, evaluation, and management of high blood pressure in adults: a report of the American College of Cardiology/American Heart Association Task Force on Clinical practice guidelines. J Am Coll Cardiol 2018;71:2239; with permission.

level to assess for cardiac injury. A urinalysis can be done to assess for proteinuria or hematuria.[19] If the cause is suspected to be drug induced, then a urine toxicology should also be performed. If the patient is a woman and pregnancy is possible, a urine or serum human chorionic gonadotropin hormone test should be obtained.[19] Patients with a hypertensive emergency should have an electrocardiogram upon presentation and routine 2-view chest radiograph.[19] If a pulmonary embolus is suspected, a CT with angiogram should be performed on the chest.[19] If there is evidence of mental status change, focal weakness, or any new abnormal neurologic findings are present, a CT of the head without contrast should also be performed.[19] For close and accurate monitoring, insertion of an arterial line should also be considered.[19]

Treatment

Once the presence of end organ damage is established, careful treatment should begin considering the patient's age, stability, and comorbidities. Because autoregulation of BP and tissue perfusion are altered, a continuous infusion of a short-acting titratable medication is recommended as first line to prevent further end organ damage.[5] The goal of intravenous antihypertensives is to minimize or stop end organ damage, identify the cause, and treat early with proper antihypertensives (**Table 5**).[5] In the specific cases of severe preeclampsia, eclampsia, or pheochromocytoma, the SBP should be immediately reduced to less than 140 mm Hg within the first hour and to less than 120 mm Hg in aortic dissection.[5] There is great risk with quickly lowering BP and may result in worsening renal, cerebral, and/or coronary ischemia, and careful patient monitoring is indicated.[5] If there is no evidence of an aortic dissection, severe preeclampsia or eclampsia, or pheochromocytoma, the recommendation is to reduce the BP by 25% over the first hour, then to 160/100 mm Hg over the next 2 to 6 hours, and then to normal over the next 24 to 48 hours.[5] Patients should be closely monitored throughout the process.

SUMMARY

A one-size-fits-all approach to managing and treating hypertension is ineffective. Collaboration and communication between patient and clinician are important aspects of achieving control of hypertension. Patient risk factors, age, ethnicity, comorbid conditions, diet, health habits, sleep patterns, current medications including the use of over-the-counter medications or supplements, willingness to participate in lifestyle modification, and BP monitoring should be taken into consideration when determining an individualized plan of care. Ensuring accuracy of BP measurement is paramount to ensure appropriateness of treatment and reduce adverse effects related to medication. An individualized, multifaceted evidence-based approach is necessary to reduce the risk of death related to CVD, stroke, and kidney disease and improve health outcomes.

REFERENCES

1. Benjamin EJ, Virani SS, Callaway CW, et al. Heart disease and stroke statistics 2018 update: a report from the American heart association. Circulation 2018; 137:e67–492.
2. Verdecchia P, Gentile G, Angeli F, et al. Influence of blood pressure reduction on composite cardiovascular endpoints in clinical trials. J Hypertens 2010;28(7): 1356–65.
3. Dominiczak AF, Kuo D. Hypertension: update 2017. Hypertension 2017;69:3–4.
4. Mozzafarian D, Benjamin EJ, Go AS, et al. Heart disease and stroke statistics-2015 update: a report from the American Heart Association. Circulation 2015; 131:e29–322.
5. Whelton PK, Carey RM, Aronow WS, et al. 2017 ACC/AHA/AAPA/ABC/ACPM/AGS/APhA/ASH/ASPC/NMA/PCNA guideline for the prevention, detection, evaluation, and management of high blood pressure in adults: a report of the American

College of Cardiology/American Heart Association Task Force on Clinical Practice Guidelines. J Am Coll Cardiol 2018;71:e127–248.

6. Chang AR, Sang Y, Leddy J, et al. Antihypertensive medications and the prevalence of hyperkalemia in a large health system. Hypertension 2016;67:1181–8.

7. Calhoun DA, Jones D, Textor S, et al. Resistant hypertension: diagnosis, evaluation, and treatment: a scientific statement from the American heart association professional education committee of the council for high blood pressure research. Hypertension 2008;51:1403–19.

8. Gradman AH, Basile JN, Carter BL, et al. Combination therapy in hypertension. J Clin Hypertens (Greenwich) 2011;13:146–54.

9. Thomopoulos C, Parati G, Zanchetti A. Effects of blood pressure lowering on outcome incidence in hypertension: 7. Effects of more vs. less intensive blood pressure lowering and different achieved blood pressure levels–updated overview and meta-analyses of randomized trials. J Hypertens 2016;34:613–22.

10. Yaxley J, Thambar S. Resistant hypertension: an approach to management in primary care. J Family Med Prim Care 2015;4(2):193–9.

11. Cohen D, Peixoto A. Hypertension. Nephrology Self-Assessment Program 2016; 15(1).

12. De Rosa M. Resistant hypertension: definition, evaluation, and new therapeutic approaches to treatment. Diseases and Disorders 2017;1(1).

13. Million Hearts. Improving medication adherence among patients with hypertension: a tip sheet for health care professionals. Available at: https://millionhearts. hhs.gov/files/TipSheet_HCP_MedAdherence.pdf. Accessed October 31, 2018.

14. Fischer MA, Choudhry NK, Brill G, et al. Trouble getting started: predictors of primary care medication nonadherence. Am J Med 2011;124(11):1089.e9–22.

15. Torun D. Approach to cases with resistant hypertension. Anadolu Kardiyol Derg 2014;14(2):192–5.

16. Bakris G, Sorrentino M. Hypertension: a companion to Braunwald's heart disease. 3rd edition. Philadelphia: Elsevier; 2018.

17. Kapur V, Auckley D, Chowdhuri S, et al. Clinical practice guideline for diagnostic testing for adult obstructive sleep apnea: an American Academy of Sleep Medicine Clinical Practice Guideline. J Clin Sleep Med 2017;13(3):479–504.

18. Borrelli S, De Nicola L, Stanzione G, et al. Resistant hypertension in nondialysis chronic kidney disease. Int J Hypertens 2013;2013:1–8.

19. Taal M, Chertow G, Marsden P, et al. Brenner and Rector's the kidney. 9th edition. Philadelphia: Elsevier; 2012.

20. Brown DF, Hirashima ET. Hypertensive Emergencies: Rosen & Barkin's five-minute emergency consult. 5th edition. Philadelphia: Wolters Kluwer Health; 2015.

21. Danaei G, Ding EL, Mozaffarian D, et al. The preventable causes of death in the United States: comparative risk assessment of dietary, lifestyle, and metabolic risk factors. PLoS Med 2009;6:e1000058.

22. Ford ES. Trends in mortality from all causes and cardiovascular disease among hypertensive and nonhypertensive adults in the United States. Circulation 2011;123:1737–44.

Culinary Medicine
Patient Education for Therapeutic Lifestyle Changes

Nanette LeBlanc-Morales, DNP, NP-C

KEYWORDS

- Culinary • Culinary medicine • Cardiovascular disease • Lifestyle medicine
- Nutrition

KEY POINTS

- Preventable chronic diseases, such as cardiovascular disease, is a growing epidemic in the United States largely related to unhealthy lifestyle behaviors and potentially delays wound healing, extends hospital stay, and increases hospital-related complications.
- Therapies targeting diet and nutrition can promote health, reduce risk factors for CVD, and reverse cardiometabolic disorders that can compound comorbidities and subsequent increased mortality in hospitalized patients.
- Culinary medicine is the application of evidence-based food science to treat and manage disease that is tailored to patient health needs and goals.
- Patients equipped with nutritional knowledge and instructed on culinary techniques can implement sustainable changes in diet behaviors that affect the course of their disease pursuant to hospital discharge.

Culinary medicine (CM) is an emerging field of evidence-based medical practice with an emphasis on healthy eating. In 2003, CM began as an elective course on cooking and nutrition at the State University of New York-Upstate Medical University. A decade later, the Goldring Center for Culinary Medicine at Tulane in New Orleans, Louisiana, was developed as an interactive program with the mission to equip medical providers and the community with skills on nutrition, meal planning, and meal preparation. The premise of CM is health promotion and illness management through calculated dietary regimens based on health needs, budget, and lifestyle. CM should not be confused with alternative medicine, herbal medicine, or naturopathic therapies. Rather, it is a taxonomy using particular dietary components of food in the context of their biologic effects on body systems. Simply put, it is the "Science of medicine blended with the art of cooking."[1]

Disclosure Statement: The author has nothing to disclose.
Graduate Program, School of Nursing, LSU Health Sciences Center – New Orleans, 1900 Gravier, New Orleans, LA 70112, USA
E-mail address: nmoral@lsuhsc.edu

CULINARY MEDICINE: A RECIPE FOR GOOD HEALTH

The philosophy of CM is based on the relationship between nutrition knowledge and application of culinary strategies that are tailored to a patient's needs. The practice of CM is not devoid of pharmaceutical management but rather places primary focus on integration of culinary knowledge and cooking personalized for an individual's skill level, budget, lifestyle, and culture. CM follows a systematic application of evidence-based food science to treat and manage a specific disease. Implementation of CM in the health care setting requires the medical provider to be well versed and trained in culinary principles. Use of this skill along with knowledge of the pathophysiologic effects of food on disease processes guide the therapeutic plan. An integral part in the practice of CM is a patient's active role in learning and implementing prescribed food regimens. Patients receive education and demonstration of how to strategically shop for a variety of foods and prepare them to manage their particular illness. CM considers socioeconomic restraints and cultural preferences in meal planning, which encourages sustainability of the diet changes. These considerations make for goal-oriented therapy that is practical and sensitive to the patient's needs. Providers facilitate behavioral changes through education and instruction. This dialogue fosters a patient's better understanding of healthy food preparation and helps alleviate perceived barriers related to cost and time. CM can treat many health conditions as evidenced in research but is especially successful in prevention and treatment of cardiovascular disease (CVD).

EPIDEMIOLOGY: CARDIOVASCULAR DISEASE

According to the World Health Organization and the Centers for Disease Control and Prevention (CDC), CVD is among the top four most common chronic diseases affecting the United States. CVD alone claims about 610,000 deaths per year in the United States.[2] Additional CDC statistics represent the magnitude of heart disease in the US population:

- Heart disease is the leading cause of death in men and women.
- In 2015, more than 50% of deaths caused by heart disease was in men.
- In 2015, a total of 366,000 people died of the most common type of CVD: coronary heart disease.
- 1 in 4 deaths is attributed to heart disease.
- Heart disease is the leading cause of death for people of most racial/ethnic groups in the United States.
- Nearly 1 million Americans suffer a heart attack each year.
- Heart disease costs the United States about $200 billion each year. This total includes the cost of health care services, medications, and lost productivity (**Fig. 1**).

PATHOPHYSIOLOGY OF CARDIOVASCULAR DISEASE

CVD is caused by disruption of biologic and physiologic processes that affect the heart and endothelium of blood vessels. The two main factors leading to CVD are hypertension (HTN) and atherosclerosis. HTN is defined as a systolic blood pressure greater than or equal to 140 and diastolic blood pressure greater than or equal to 90. This is caused by either a genetic predisposition, lifestyle, or both. A poor diet high in sodium, tobacco use, obesity, and insulin resistance are all risk factors in the development of HTN. High blood pressure overloads the heart and with time cardiac muscle becomes scarred and weak and less efficient. Blood flow is compromised

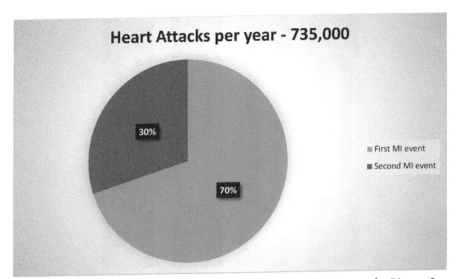

Fig. 1. Heart attacks per year. MI, myocardial infarction. (*Data from* Centers for Disease Control and Prevention, National Center for Health Statistics. Multiple cause of death 1999–2015. CDC WONDER online database. Available at: http://wonder.cdc.gov/mcd-icd10.html. Accessed August 10, 2018.)

and the heart is no longer able to deliver much needed oxygen and nutrients to cells adequately. There is synergistic insult to the lining of blood vessels through inflammation and plaque formation called atherosclerosis. Inflammation initiates the sequela of lipid accumulation in the vessel wall, fatty lesions, and fibrotic plaque. The build-up of plaque in vasculature causes a narrowing of the blood vessel lumen and further inhibits blood flow. This lack of oxygen and nutrient transport leads to progressive deterioration of cardiovascular (CV) function. Complications that occur as a result of untreated CVD include thrombosis, angina, myocardial infarction (MI), heart failure, stroke, aortic aneurysm, and peripheral artery disease, all of which contribute to the morbidity and mortality in those with CVD (**Fig. 2**).

RISK FACTORS

CVD is a preventable disease directly related to lifestyle habits, such as diet and physical activity. Some individuals are more likely to develop CVD, such as those with metabolic syndrome (MetS). Diagnosis of MetS requires three or more of the following:

- Waist circumference >102 cm for men and >88 cm for women
- Triglyceride level >150 mg/dL
- High-density lipoprotein cholesterol <40 mg/dL in men or <50 mg/dL in women
- Systolic blood pressure >130 mm Hg or diastolic blood pressure >85 mm Hg
- Fasting plasma glucose >110 mg/dL

Additional risk factors include high blood pressure, hyperlipidemia, smoking, diabetes, obesity, and excessive alcohol intake. According to the CDC, almost 50% of Americans have at least three or more risk factors for CVD.[2] Measures to modify risk factors that contribute to the development of heart disease would have an impact on associated morbidity and mortality, especially for hospitalized patients in a critical care setting. These patients must increase energy expenditure to support the immune

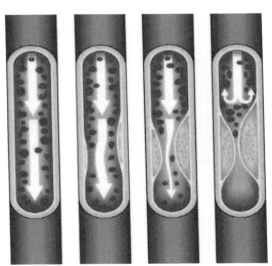

Fig. 2. Plaque formation. (*Data from* Centers for Disease Control and Prevention. Heart disease facts. Available at: http://cdc.gov/heart disease/facts.htm. Accessed August 10, 2018.)

response and compensatory organ function, which taxes the biologic process in critically ill individuals. CM uses nutritional education and directives aimed at changing unhealthy eating habits, such as consuming a diet high in fat, by empowering an individual to make better choices. A person taught dietary basics along with culinary counseling is better equipped to engage in preventative eating habits whereby decreasing risk of chronic illnesses, such as CVD, and increasing a hospitalized patient's reserve for healing and maintenance of normal physiologic function in an already vulnerable state.

IMPLICATIONS OF CULINARY MEDICINE IN MANAGEMENT OF CARDIOVASCULAR DISEASE

It is widely acknowledged that healthy lifestyles that include physical exercise, good food choices, and psychosocial well-being contribute to prevention of numerous debilitating diseases. This knowledge has led to an increased interest in integrative or complimentary medical therapies to treat chronic illnesses, such as CVD. Robust research shows that a consistent diet of fruits, vegetables, and low-fat proteins can improve or even resolve high blood pressure, dyslipidemia, diabetes mellitus, and obesity but the benefits of dietary interventions go beyond the containment of a particular disease.[3,4] The benefits of dietary interventions also reduces the prevalence of comorbidities associated with CVD (eg, peripheral artery disease, heart failure, MI, renal insufficiency, and stroke).[5] The positive outcomes of healthy lifestyle choices in chronic disease is evident in CM practice with reduced incidence of morbidity and mortality associated with untreated CVD.[6,7] CM also promotes a high quality of life.[8] Conventional medicine with the use of pharmaceuticals, although effective, is not without risks. Patients with CVD are on multiple medications for management placing them at risk for complications associated with polypharmacy. Furthermore, the cost of medication is a barrier to compliance for many patients ultimately leading to worsening CVD and associated complications. Treatment modalities that use behavioral modification for primary intervention of preventable diseases can decrease the risk of complications, improve quality of life, and contain health care cost related to conventional treatments.

THE CASE FOR FUNCTIONAL FOOD
Mediterranean Diet

A plant-based diet, also referred to as a Mediterranean diet, has multiple health benefits on a metabolic and physiologic level that help the body function optimally and fight disease. Fruits and vegetables are rich in vitamins and antioxidants that promote health and improve complications in CVD. Antioxidants prevent oxidative stress, which is a mediator of endothelial inflammation. Those that consume diets high in a variety of green leafy vegetables with limited intake of fat and refined sugars are less likely to be overweight. In addition, green leafy vegetables contain vitamin K, an essential element in the prevention of atherosclerosis. The Mediterranean diet also reduces the risk of other chronic diseases, such as diabetes mellitus and obesity, risk factors for coronary heart disease. Diets rich in a variety of fruits can lower the risk of diabetes by at least 12%.[9] Individuals diagnosed with diabetes can expect a 13% to 18% risk reduction in mortality and/or subsequent development of complications including microvascular and macrovascular disease that affects the kidneys, eyes, and nerves.[10]

DASH Diet

The DASH diet is endorsed by the American Heart Association (AHA) and the National Institutes of Medicine for the treatment of high blood pressure.[11] It is a reliable source of potassium, magnesium, and calcium, which are essential in heart health. The main elements in this diet include a salt restriction of 1500 to 2300 mg per day and low-fat/high-fiber food choices, such as whole grains. This modified "Western" diet helps to lower blood pressure and cholesterol. It also decreases the risk of cancer, stroke, and heart disease. An additional benefit of the DASH diet is that it induces weight loss, which in turn improves/prevents MetS, a precursor to CVD.

Vegetarian Diet

There are several variations to the vegetarian diet. The primary differences among them is the inclusion or avoidance of flesh foods, dairy, or eggs. Regardless of the food groups consumed, the vegetarian diet offers health benefits in the primary prevention of disease and management of modifiable chronic diseases. Expected outcomes when following the vegetarian diet are lower body mass index (BMI), improved insulin sensitivity, and decreased cholesterol. It is considered superior to diets that allow consumption of meat, poultry, and fish in the management of obesity.[9,11] The most significant benefit of a vegetarian diet, however, is in the prevention of risk factors leading to CVD but are amenable to a healthier diet. CVD risk factors include HTN, dyslipidemia, elevated blood glucose serum levels, and atherosclerotic plaque.

Anti-inflammatory Diet

Anti-inflammatory diets are considered "low-energy diets"[12] characterized by decreased intake of saturated fats and refined carbohydrates while increasing foods containing antioxidants and omega-3 fatty acids. Compounds are found in such foods as herbs, spices, fish, and fruits, which aid in modulation of the autoimmune responses leading to inflammation in chronic illnesses, such as arthritis and multiple sclerosis. Leafy greens, such as spinach, kale, broccoli, and cabbage, contain vitamin K, which also plays an important role in the inflammatory pathway.

EVIDENCE-BASED USE OF HERBS, SPICES, AND VITAMINS

Human survival depends on consumption of basic nutrients but food is more than just a source of energy and essential vitamins and minerals. Since prehistoric times, food has been known to have medicinal properties (**Table 1**). Phytochemicals are compounds found in various fruits, vegetables, grains, and other plants that treat diseases, promote healing, and maintain protective biologic activity.

Ginger

Ginger is a flowering plant that research has shown to be used as a safe natural remedy for postoperative and pregnancy-induced nausea.[13,14] It is usually used as a culinary spice easily found in local supermarkets and in pharmacies as an over-the-counter supplement. It can also be considered for treatment of pain and swelling in those with osteoarthritis.[15]

Oregano

Oregano is an herb used as a condiment or spice. It is a common seasoning in Mediterranean dishes and has long been used for pharmacologic remedies. It is known to have antimicrobial properties against food-borne pathogens, it contains antioxidants that offer CV and nervous system protection, it helps in regulation of blood sugar and lipids, and has anti-inflammatory effects.[16]

Basil

Substantive data highlight the positive effects that basil has on metabolic disorders, memory and cognition, immunity and inflammation, and skin health. It is found in many cosmetic products, such as shampoo, lotions, facial masks, and soaps because of dermatologic benefits. In randomized trials it was also shown to treat gingivitis and reduce the level of oral bacteria, such as *Streptococcus mutans*.[17]

Vitamin D

Vitamin D is a fat-soluble vitamin that is found in a limited number of foods. It is often an additive in food products, such as dairy. The major source of vitamin D is sunlight exposure but can also be taken as a supplement. Bone health is dependent on optimal

Table 1
Recommended diets for chronic conditions

Chronic Condition	Recommended Diet/Food
Rheumatoid arthritis	Anti-inflammatory diet[28]
Epilepsy	Ketogenic diet[24]
CVD	Mediterranean diet[30]
Colon cancer	Mediterranean diet[31]
Type II diabetes mellitus	Mediterranean diet[32]
Hypertension	Soy nuts[33]
Hyperlipidemia	Legumes[34]
Metabolic syndrome	Tree nuts[35]
Heart failure	Baked/broiled fish[36]
Acute cough	Honey and milk[37]

Data from Refs.[28–37]

serum levels. It also plays a ... intake of vitamin D puts one at ris... diac arrhythmias. The incidence of ...tion of cancer and diabetes. Insufficient vitamin D deficiency. One study shov...e healing, osteoporosis, and even car- was associated with increased risk of dea...actor for CVD, is inversely related to the neurovascular protective value and pote...ow serum vitamin D (<30 ng/mL) ...ry to stroke.[18] This underscores ...vent CVD.

Garlic

Garlic is commonly used as a flavorful additive in rec... concentration is the mechanism of action by which age...ulation of adiponectin and prevent CVD. Adiponectin is a hormone that has direc... extract helps treat production and is necessary for healthy endothelial function... on nitrous oxide garlic can reduce blood pressure by as much as 9 to 16 mm Hg ar...dies show that cholesterol.[20] Garlic has also shown to cause a reduction in C-reactive...rease serum flammatory marker that is an indication of atherosclerosis. ...tein, an in-

PATIENT EDUCATION

The ideal application of CM is in primary prevention of chronic disease. The 2010 American College of Cardiology Foundation/AHA report on assessment of CV risk states that adult women and men should receive global risk scoring and family history of CVD should be noted for CV risk assessment.[21] Patients need to be made aware of the importance of regular health visits to their primary care provider (PCP) for CVD screening. Family history, especially a history of early onset CVD, can direct early primary preventative measures. The customary postdischarge follow-up with a PCP is imperative where continued culinary management will be reinforced. Nursing providers are also expected to include dietary instruction in discharge planning for secondary and tertiary prevention. Nursing interventions that include education on significance of social history, such as tobacco use or alcohol consumption, as it relates to CVD risk may help discourage these behaviors. Geriatric patients are at particular risk because there is a characteristic increased prevalence of risk factors for CVD, such as HTN, dyslipidemia, and glucose intolerance. The nurse can encourage patients to self-monitor blood pressure because HTN is mostly an asymptomatic condition. Diabetes mellitus is also frequently asymptomatic. Providers should instruct the patient on common symptoms that need to be reported to one's PCP including unusual fatigue, increased thirst or hunger, and increased urination. Special populations that are at higher risk for development of CVD including women and minority ethnicities, such as blacks or African Americans and nonwhite Hispanics should be informed of their added risk and need for disease prevention. Women are slightly more likely to develop HTN than men, especially those of postmenopausal age.[22] Patient education generates awareness and increases the likelihood of self-care measures. Critical care nurses have an integral role in bridging the gap between patient knowledge and patient action.

Culinary Medicine in Primary Prevention

Patients should understand the benefits of healthy eating include the reduction of risk of coronary heart disease and in treatment of diagnosed heart disease. CM promotes a diet that is rich in vitamins and nutrients that are protective for the CV system and promote health. Antioxidants, omega-3 fatty acids, fiber, unsaturated fats, vitamin D, and vitamin K are found in the Mediterranean diet, which includes a variety of fresh fruits, vegetables, whole grains, fish, and lean beef or pork. Cooking meals seasoned

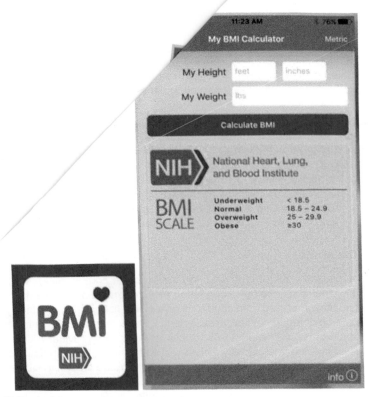

Fig. 3. BMI calculator.

with garlic could be one approach to help lower cholesterol. A daily dose of garlic modestly lowers cholesterol by as much as 7% and may lower blood pressure[20] and inhibit platelet aggregation.[23] Fast food and processed foods should avoided because they are usually high in sodium. The US Department of Health and Human Services 2015 to 2020 dietary guidelines recommend less than 2300 mg/d of sodium daily.[24] Execution of CM includes patient teaching on how to read and interpret food labels, which is a source of information regarding the nutritional value of the food item. Terms to recognize are *trans*-fat, saturated fat, and hydrogenated fat, which are all unhealthy fats that should be avoided. Although CM is directed toward nutritional coaching, patients are also encouraged to engage in moderate exercise daily or weekly as tolerated. This helps reduce CV risk associated with obesity. It also boosts metabolism, prompts weight loss, and strengthens the CV system. A healthy weight reduces the risk of HTN and MetS, both risk factors for CVD. BMI is a helpful tool that calculates an individual's recommended weight (**Fig. 3**). Patients can download the BMI calculator from the US Department of Health and Human Services Web site to their cellphone. Other recommendations include smoke cessation and alcohol in moderation.

In summary

- Avoid high-calorie/low-nutrition foods (sugary beverages, candy)
- Consume a variety of fruits, vegetables, legumes, nuts, low-fat dairy, whole grains
- Use oils low in saturated fat (canola, soybean, avocado, olive, sesame)

- Limit saturated fats and *trans*-fats (red meat, whole milk, pastries)
- No more than one to two alcoholic drinks daily
- Limit sodium intake to less than 2400 mg/d

Secondary Prevention

Medical conditions that pose a risk for development of CVD, such as MetS, should be regularly monitored and treated aggressively to avoid debilitating consequences of CV or metabolic disease. Treatment may include a combination of pharmacologic and culinary therapies. Secondary prevention is aimed at modifying or eliminating existing risk factors that can lead to complications of CVD including MI, heart failure, PAD, renal disease, and stroke. The 2011 AHA/American College of Cardiology Foundation update offers therapy guidelines for patients with atherosclerotic vascular disease (Fig. 4).[21]

CM addresses those components that contribute to this increased risk of untoward events: blood pressure, lipids, glucose intolerance or diabetes, and weight. Goals and treatment are based on a diet structure that targets specific diseases, health needs, and body function. Individuals with added risk for CV and those with existing atherosclerotic disease benefit from a Mediterranean diet in conjunction with the DASH diet. Research studies have supported this recommendation for decades but creative instruction that is tailored to each patient's health requirements, socioeconomic status, and lifestyle guides CM practice that also provides direction on cooking techniques and functional use of condiments and seasonings. Garlic is a valuable staple because it has shown to lower cholesterol and blood pressure and inhibit platelet

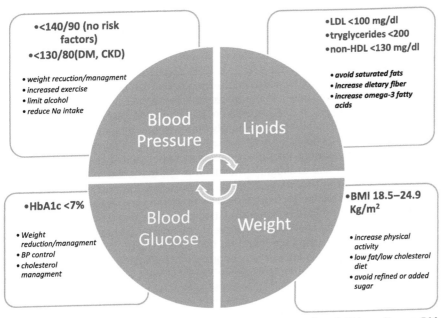

Fig. 4. Therapy guidelines and lifestyle recommendations. CKD, chronic kidney disease; DM, diabetes mellitus; HbA_{1c}, hemoglobin A_{1c}; HDL, high-density lipoprotein; LDL, low-density lipoprotein. (*Data from* Smith SC, Benjamin EJ, Bonow RO, et al. AHA/ACCF secondary prevention and risk reduction therapy for patients with coronary and other atherosclerotic vascular disease: 2011 update, a guide from the American Heart Association and American College of Cardiology Foundation. Circulation 2011;124(22):2458–73.)

aggregation.[19,20] The benefits of vitamin K found in green leafy vegetables are vaso-dilation and reduction of renal reabsorption of sodium.[4] Another positive impact is on thrombosis formation.[21] Patients with HTN are therefore encouraged to include vegetables, such as cabbage, broccoli, and greens, in their daily diet. Vegetables are mainstay of the Mediterranean diet that are rich in phytochemicals and antioxi-dants, which lowers circulatory disease mortality and cerebral vascular disease. Inflammation is one of the primary catalysts for the formation of vascular plague and is minimized by a diet that includes sources of omega 3 fatty acids and fiber. Fish is a common source of omega-3 fatty acids. Fiber is obtained from various sour-ces, such as grains, fruits, and vegetables. Antioxidants found in fruits support and protect endothelial function.[25] Berries, grapes, cabbage, legumes, chocolate, and pears all contain antioxidants. When cooking, oils low in saturated fats, such as canola, olive, sesame, soybean, and avocado are recommended over vegetable oil. CM medicine does not simply advocate for healthy eating by a balanced diet incorpo-rating all food groups. It is a deliberate and concise plan specific to the medical con-dition through general principles of a primary and secondary preventative diet:

- Reduce the intake of saturated fats, *trans*-fats, and cholesterol
- Increase portions of fruits and vegetables relative to proteins
- Proteins should be lean cuts (eg, pork loin, beef round/loin, beef choice, or select)
- Ensure adequate viscous fiber
- Omega-3 fatty acids (**Table 2**)

Implementation of Culinary Medicine: A Prescription for FOOD

Food can be prescribed in a similar format to how medications are prescribed. Dr LaPuma, considered the pioneer of CM, suggests a structure using the acronym FOOD (**Box 1**).

Shopping

Grocery shopping for a prescribed food regimen can be overwhelming. Patients equipped with the skills to navigate the grocery market can easily locate the necessary items within their budget. In CM, patients are taught how to determine and compare the value of similar items to maximize quality and quantity of foods purchased. Such tips as buying in bulk, choosing fruits that are in season, and consideration of more economical options, such as frozen vegetables as opposed to fresh vegetables, can help the patient feel more confident in their shopping experience. When an individual experiences comfort in this process they are more likely to continue the pattern of practical grocery shopping. Patients are guided through this process starting with a meal plan based on the food prescription. The next step is menu planning, which en-tails listing needed ingredients and building a shopping list. Easy to follow handouts to help organize food shopping are found on the CM Web site (culinarymedicine.org). Planning ahead saves time and makes shopping more efficient. Leah Sarris, Program Director for the Goldring Center for Culinary Medicine, recommends that when shop-ping, one should spend most of the time in the parameter of the market because this is generally where the healthiest foods are located. Also, grouping food items to location in the store can optimize one's time. Patients are also coached on assessing produce by observing color, texture, symmetry, and aroma.

Preparing

In CM practice it may be useful to share with patients that when preparing prescribed food consider multiple uses for a food item that can reduce waste, save money, and

Table 2
Risk factor and food prescription

Risk Factor	Recommended Goals	Food Prescription
Hypertension	<140/90, <130/80 with history of DM or CKD	Mediterranean diet + DASH diet Avoid caffeine Cook with sesame oil Add cocoa for flavor Drinking mineral water Soy nuts Season dishes with garlic
Hyperlipidemia	LDL <100 Triglycerides <200 Non-HDL-C <130	Nuts (almonds, hazelnuts) Avocados as fruit choice and/or Avocado oil for cooking Flax meal, cinnamon as condiment Soy milk Salmon, tuna Season dishes with garlic
Glucose intolerance/ diabetes	HbA$_{1c}$ <7%	Mediterranean diet Eating structure and timing: eat at consistent intervals throughout the day
Overweight/obese	BMI 18.5–24.9	Increased dietary fiber: flax seed meal, steel cut oats, quinoa Sprouted grain bread in replacement of whole-grain bread Berries, apples

Abbreviations: CKD, chronic kidney disease; DM, diabetes mellitus; HbA$_{1c}$, hemoglobin A$_{1c}$; HDL-C, high-density lipoprotein cholesterol; LDL, low-density lipoprotein.

offer additional nutritional benefits. For instance, when preparing vegetables for cooking every part of the food item has utility. Although the stalk of a carrot or celery may be prepared for seasoning, the leaves that are usually wasted can be used for making a vegetable stock or chopped and used as a topping for salads. Broccoli stems can also be used in vegetable stock. This is ideal for those that need to decrease dietary sodium because many store-bought stocks contain large amounts of salt. Many patients do not appreciate the versatility of food items that also accommodate a modest budget.

Box 1
Food prescription

- Frequency: refers to how often the particular food or meal should be eaten
- Objective: what is the intended goal of the food or diet? (weight loss, health)
- Options: describes meal planning, budgeting, shopping, food preparation, which can be tailored to the patient's specific needs or limitations
- Duration: the time scale of the food or meal to be eaten (daily, weekly, monthly)

Cooking

Instruction on cooking techniques is arguably the most important step in the practice of CM. This involves a deliberate pairing of food, herbs, and spices to balance flavor with healthy eating. If healthy food does not taste good then patients are not likely to maintain the prescribed diet. Salt generally enhances flavor in dishes but for those with HTN added sodium must be avoided. Patients are taught what staples to keep stocked in their pantry that can aggrandize tastefulness but preserve the intended nutritional value of the dish to meet the need of the patient's condition. Healthier substitutes that can be used are onions, garlic, and pepper, which are considered aromatics. Garlic has additional phytonutrients that specifically aid in management of CVD. Herbs, such as oregano and basil, are also good choices to augment disease-modifying benefits in CVD. Vinegars, wine, and citrus, such as lemons or limes, are additional savory options. To reduce fat content especially found in baked goods, one can remove oils and lard and replace it with mashed bananas, unsweetened applesauce, or even yogurt. Certain cooking oils provide omega-3 fatty acids, which is beneficial for those with CVD, such as olive oil, canola oil, and flaxseed oil. These are preferred over other oils, such as corn or vegetable. Even cooking temperatures can affect the amount of antioxidants important for endothelial function.[26,27]

Sustaining Changes Through Technology

The dialogue between medical provider and patient in the practice of CM provides instructional guidance that the patient can use day-to-day but also provides patients with knowledge and resources to continue their illness-directed healthy lifestyle. Use of traditional education methods combined with technology can help support patients when outside of the clinic examination room. A plethora of World Wide Web–based programs and mobile applications are tools that patients can use to assess baseline health status to guide health goals. There are meal trackers that keep track of meals including such data as calories, fat, carbohydrates, and proteins. Fitness applications record physical activity and in some cases calories burned. The ultimate goal of CM practice is for the patient to sustain healthy eating habits and change the course of their disease or reduce risk of illness. Integration of World Wide Web–based and mobile programs empower and engages patients in the process toward optimal health. These programs are generally user friendly and obtained free of charge. National health organizations, such as the CDC and AHA, have additional resources for patients that can be accessed and used in their diet plan of care.

SUMMARY

Chronic disease continues to plague the United States partly because of an aging population with a longer life expectancy. However, lifestyle behavior is recognized as the central catalyst in development of many preventable chronic illness. A healthy diet and physical activity help reduce risk factors leading to debilitating conditions, such as CVD. Pharmaceuticals treat diseases but can also complicate the primary health condition. Behavioral change therapies to treat or prevent chronic illness are effective and reduce health care cost while engaging the patient to invest in their own health. CM is a clinical discipline that is based on scientific evidence using nutritional interventions to meet the purpose of health maintenance, health promotion, and disease prevention. It is a collaborative partnership structured to teach patients how nutrition relates to health and how to use culinary techniques to maximize the therapeutic effects of food. Affecting changes in dietary behavior achieves the desired outcome of CM: a sustainable dietary lifestyle leading to health and well-being.

Despite decades of validated research on th... of a healthy diet, CM remains a fairly recent development in formal medical p... rm evidence connects delib- erate dietary choices to targeted health conditio... rms the foundation of non- medicinal therapy, but studies on illness-directed... management are lacking. Further investigation of culinary interventions is n... address the growing disparity between health knowledge and patient mana... Nurses serve as pa- tient advocates in the form of patient education and cou... ion of care. There is often a disconnect between clinical information and patient u... tanding. Instruction on culinary concepts can deflect patient confusion and promo... erence to dietary plan. This sets the tone for patient behavior outside the hospital... g to avoid read- mission, improve quality of life, and extend years of life.

REFERENCES

1. LaPuma J. What is culinary medicine and what does it do? Popul Health Manag 2016;19(1):1–3.
2. Heart disease facts. Centers for Disease Control and Prevention. CDC website. Available at: http://cdc.gov/heart disease/facts.htm. Accessed August 10, 2018.
3. Yokoyama Y, Nishimura K, Barnard ND, et al. Vegetarian diets and blood pressure: a meta-analysis. JAMA Intern Med 2014;174(4):577–87.
4. Franz MJ, Boucher JL, Rutten-Ramos S, et al. Lifestyle weight-loss intervention outcomes in overweight and obese adults with type 2 diabetes: a systematic review and meta-analysis of randomized clinical trials. J Acad Nutr Diet 2015; 115(9):1447–63.
5. de Lorgeril M, Salen P, Martin JL, et al. Effect of a Mediterranean type of diet on the rate of cardiovascular complications in patients with coronary artery disease insights into the cardioprotective effect of certain nutriments. J Am Coll Cardiol 1996;28(5):1103–8.
6. Restrepo BJ, Rieger M. Trans fat and cardiovascular disease mortality: evidence from bans in restaurants in New York. J Health Econ 2016;45:176–96.
7. Micha R, Peñalvo JL, Cudhea F, et al. Association between dietary factors and mortality from heart disease, stroke, and type 2 diabetes in the United States. JAMA 2017;317(9):912–24.
8. Evans J, Magee A, Dickman K, et al. A plant-based nutrition program: nurses experience the benefits and challenges of following a plant-based diet. Am J Nurs 2017;17(3):56–61.
9. Melina V, Winston C, Levin S. Position of the academy of nutrition and dietetics: vegetarian diets. J Acad Nutr Diet 2012;116(12):1970–80.
10. Du H, Li L, Bennett D, et al. Fresh fruit consumption in relation to incident diabetes and diabetic vascular complications: a 7-y prospective study of .5 million Chinese adults. PLoS Med 2017;14(4):e1002279. Available at: https://doi.org/10.1371/journal. pmed.1002279.
11. Your guide to lowering blood pressure. US Department of Health and Human Services. National Institutes of Health Web site. Available at: https://www.nhlbi.nih.gov/files/docs/public/heart/hbp_low.pdf. Accessed August 19, 2018.
12. Labuschagne IL, Blaauw R. An anti-inflammatory approach to the dietary management of multiple sclerosis: a condensed review. South Afr J Clin Nutr 2018; 31(3):67–73.
13. White B. Ginger: an overview. Am Fam Physician 2007;75(11):1689–91.
14. Jewell D, Young G. Interventions for nausea and vomiting in early pregnancy. Cochrane Database Syst Rev 2003;(4):CD000145.

15. Therkleson T. Ginger c ... therapy for adults with osteoarthritis. J Adv Nurs 2010;66(10):2225–33.

16. Singletary KW. Oreg ... rview of the literature on health benefits. Nutr Today 2010;45(3):129–39.

17. Singletary KW. B ... brief summary of potential health benefits. Nutr Today 2018;53(2):92–7.

18. Sheerah HA, B ...S, Cui R, et al. Relationship between dietary vitamin D and ... and coronary heart disease: the Japan collaborative cohort ... deaths from 18;49(2):454–7. study. Stro

19. Patricio L ...e role of adiponectin in cardiometabolic diseases: effects of nutritional int ...ntions. J Nutr 2016;146(suppl):422S–6S.

20. Ravi V ...thew JB. Garlic and heart disease. J Nutr 2016;146(Suppl):416S–21S.

21. AHA/A ...CF secondary prevention and risk reduction therapy for patients with coronary and other atherosclerotic vascular disease: 2011 update: a guideline from the American heart Association and American College of Cardiology Foundation. Circulation 2011;124(22):2458–73.

22. Risks for heart disease and stroke. Million Hearts. U.S. Department of Health and Human Services, CDC Web site. Available at: https://millionhearts.hhs.gov/learn-prevent/risks.htm. Accessed August 19, 2018.

23. Khalid R, Gordon ML, Sarah S. Aged garlic extract inhibits human platelet aggregation by altering intracellular signaling and platelet shape change. J Nutr 2016; 146(2):410S–5S.

24. Dietary Guidelines for Americans 2015-2020. 8th edition. U.S. Department of Health and Human Services, U.S. Department of Agriculture. CDC Website. Available at: https://health/gov/dietaryguidelines/2015resources/2015-2020_Dietary_Guidelines.pdf. Accessed August 19, 2018.

25. Esposito K, Marfella R, Ciotola M, et al. Effect of a Mediterranean-style diet on endothelial dysfunction and markers of vascular inflammation in the metabolic syndrome: a randomized trial. JAMA 2004;292(12):1440–6.

26. LaPuma J. Chef MD's big book of culinary medicine. New York: Three Rivers Press; 2008.

27. Sexson K, Lindauer A, Harvath T. Supporting family caregivers: no longer home alone. AJN 2017;117(5):58–60.

28. Adam O, Beringer C, Kless T, et al. Anti-inflammatory effects of a low arachidonic acid diet and fish oil in patients with rheumatoid arthritis. Rheumatol Int 2003; 23(1):27–36.

29. Levy RG, Cooper PN, Giri P. Ketogenic diet and other dietary treatments for epilepsy. Cochrane Database Syst Rev 2012;(3):CD001903.

30. Estruch R, Ros E, Salas-Salvado J, et al. Primary prevention of cardiovascular disease with a Mediterranean diet. N Engl J Med 2013;368:1279–90.

31. Meyerhardt JA, Neidzwiecki D, Hollis D, et al. Association of dietary pattern with cancer recurrence and survival in patients with stage III colon cancer. JAMA 2007;298:754–64.

32. Koloverou E, Esposito K, Giugliano D, et al. The effect of Mediterranean diet on the development of type 2 diabetes mellitus: a meta-analysis of 10 prospective studies and 136,846 participants. Metabolism 2014;63:903–11.

33. Welty FK, Lee KS, Lew NS, et al. Effect of soy nuts on blood pressure and lipid levels in hypertensive, pre-hypertensive, and normotensive post-menopausal women. Arch Intern Med 2007;167:1060–7.

34. Ha V, Sievenpiper JL, de Souza RJ, et al. Effect of dietary pulse intake on established therapeutic lipid targets for cardiovascular risk reduction: a systematic

review and meta-analysis of randomized controlled trials. CMAJ 2014;186(8): E252–62.

35. Blanco MS. Effect of tree nuts on metabolic syndrome criteria: a systematic review and meta-analysis of randomized controlled trials. BMJ Open 2014;4(7): e004660.

36. Belin RJ, Greenland P, Martin L, et al. Fish intake and the risk of incident heart failure: the Women's Health Initiative. Circ Heart Fail 2011;4:404–13.

37. Miceli Sopo S, Greco M, Monaco S, et al. Effect of multiple honey doses on nonspecific acute cough in children: an open randomized study and literature review. Allergol Immunopathol (Madr) 2015. https://doi.org/10.1016/j.aller.2014.06.002.

Moving?

Make sure your subscription moves with you!

To notify us of your new address, find your **Clinics Account Number** (located on your mailing label above your name), and contact customer service at:

Email: journalscustomerservice-usa@elsevier.com

800-654-2452 (subscribers in the U.S. & Canada)
314-447-8871 (subscribers outside of the U.S. & Canada)

Fax number: 314-447-8029

Elsevier Health Sciences Division
Subscription Customer Service
3251 Riverport Lane
Maryland Heights, MO 63043

*To ensure uninterrupted delivery of your subscription, please notify us at least 4 weeks in advance of move.

Printed and bound by CPI Group (UK) Ltd, Croydon, CR0 4YY

03/10/2024

01040391-0010